Handbook of
Ophthalmologic
Emergencies

second edition

A GUIDE FOR EMERGENCIES IN OPHTHALMOLOGY

Y 10 5

by

GEORGE M. GOMBOS, M.D., F.A.C.S.

Professor of Ophthalmology

State University of New York

Downstate Medical Center

Brooklyn, New York

Chief of Ophthalmology

Brooklyn-Cumberland Medical Center

Brooklyn, New York

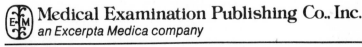

Medical Examination Publishing Co., Inc.
an Excerpta Medica company

969 Stewart Avenue • Garden City, New York 11530

notice

The editor(s) and/or author(s) and the publisher of this book have made every effort to ensure that all therapeutic modalities that are recommended are in accordance with accepted standards at the time of publication.

The drugs specified within this book may not have specific approval by the Food and Drug Administration in regard to the indications and dosages that are recommended by the editor(s) and/or author(s). The manufacturer's package insert is the best source of current prescribing information.

Copyright © 1977 by
MEDICAL EXAMINATION
PUBLISHING CO., INC.

Library of Congress Card Number
76-62573

ISBN 0-87488-633-3

July, 1977

Printed in the United States of America

Preface To The Second Edition

The great demand for this manual has made it possible to revise it in a relatively short time after its initial publication. This is an expanded edition. The previous text is revised and the bibliography is updated, but the basic format of the book remains unchanged. Despite constant changes in the choice of clinical approaches and medications, we tried to remain conservative and to describe well-accepted and practical methods of the diagnosis and treatment of ophthalmologic emergencies.

I hope that this book will remain an important source for guidance and assistance to the residents in ophthalmology, to emergency room physicians, and, in limited aspect, to paramedical personnel.

George M. Gombos

Contributors

PETER H. BALLEN, M.D., F.A.C.S.: (Trauma of the Eyelid, Orbit and Adnexa), *Professor of Clinical Ophthalmology,* State University of New York, Stony Brook, New York.

GEORGE HERMAN, M.D., F.A.C.R.: (Radiology of Ophthalmologic Emergencies), *Assistant Professor,* Mount Sinai School of Medicine, New York, New York.

RICHARD C. TROUTMAN, M.D., F.A.C.S.: (Non-Penetrating and Penetrating Injuries of the Anterior Segment), *Professor and Head of Division of Ophthalmology,* State University of New York, Downstate Medical Center, Brooklyn, New York. *Surgeon Director,* Manhattan Eye, Ear and Throat Hospital, New York, New York.

ARTHUR H. WOLINTZ, M.D., F.A.C.S.: (Neuro-Ophthalmologic Emergencies), *Associate Professor of Ophthalmology,* State University of New York, Downstate Medical Center, Brooklyn, New York. *Chief,* Division of Neuro-Ophthalmology and Ophthalmology, Kingsbrook Jewish Medical Center, Brooklyn, New York.

Foreword

It is a privilege to be asked to write the Foreword to this excellent handbook on emergency procedures for ophthalmology. This book, I believe, fills a need and, hopefully, will contribute to the prevention of unnecessary blindness as a result of traumatic injury to the eye.

The average emergency room physician or technician, though well versed in the management of acute injuries to other parts of the body, has little training or reference in the management of ocular emergencies. Also, one of the first assignments of the ophthalmic resident when he enters ophthalmology is often emergency room duty. Though a senior resident or staff ophthalmologist may be available to him, he must often make decisions well beyond his experience, and it is hoped that this handbook will also be helpful to him. To the nonophthalmologic physician, it will seem that parts of this handbook will go into greater depth in emergency management than would be necessary for him to know. This, however, is intentional since the authors have felt it necessary for the nonophthalmologist, as well as the ophthalmologist reading this volume, to understand the intricacies of definitive care of ocular injuries. Certainly it will become readily evident that advanced training is necessary to carry out these procedures, but the emergency physician should know the basis of surgical care.

The editor of this volume, Dr. George Gombos, could not be better qualified for assembling such a volume. He has been daily in contact with emergency care since the beginning of his ophthalmologic experience and, among other things, served as an emergency military ophthalmologist in the 6-day war in Israel in 1967. In addition, he has contributed to the ophthalmologic literature by detailing his experience in emergency war injuries. It is thus that I commend you to this volume in the hope that it may help both you and your patient survive the ultimate care of blindness.

Richard C. Troutman, M.D.

Acknowledgements

EDITORIAL ASSISTANCE
Aurora C. Clahane, M.S.

TECHNICAL ASSISTANCE
Doris Druce

ILLUSTRATIONS AND PHOTOGRAPHY EXECUTED BY
Department of Medical Illustration and Photography
State University of New York
Downstate Medical Center

ILLUSTRATIONS
Elizabeth Cuzzort
Associate Medical Illustrator-Photographer

Wilbert F. Davis
Senior Medical Illustrator

PHOTOGRAPHY
Willy Kratil
Supervisor of Photography

Shirley Sharf

Elisabeth White

HANDBOOK OF OPHTHALMOLOGIC EMERGENCIES

Second Edition

contents

CONTENTS (Continued)

CHAPTER 1

EYE EXAMINATION

The routine emergency-room examination of the patient with an eye problem should include the following:

> I. History
> II. Physical Examination
> III. Special Examinations

I. HISTORY: Careful history, including general information, is very important in an attempt to reach the correct diagnosis and provide appropriate treatment.

Routine questions, such as the patient's age and general health, should not be neglected under any circumstances. Very often, these questions may lead to useful information. To summarize briefly, the physician should be informed about the following:

> A. Age
> B. Occupation
> C. General health
> D. In case of accident, brief history of the accident
> E. Allergies to drugs and immunization against tetanus
> F. Condition of the eyes prior to the present illness or injury
> G. Previous eye diseases and operations

Important information may lead more quickly and more easily to the etiology of the disease or, in the case of an accident, the seriousness of the injury, and can help to provide properly administered and effective treatment.

The second part of the history should be directed to the present condition of the eye. The physician requires the following information:

> A. If the vision impaired?
> B. Is diplopia present?
> C. Is there any pain or discomfort?
> D. Is there any discharge or secretion?

After the above questions have been answered, the physician may start the physical examination of the eye.

II. PHYSICAL EXAMINATION: Physical examination of the eye should include the following:

> 1. Visual acuity
> 2. Inspection of the external ocular structures including eyelids and lacrimal apparatus
> 3. Position of the eye and eye movements

4. Pupils
5. Intraocular pressure
6. Visual fields
7. Funduscopy

VISUAL ACUITY

The most important single test of ocular function is the evaluation of visual acuity. This examination should be an integral part of the eye examination of all patients who are able to give reliable subjective responses.

Various types of letter charts are available to examine visual acuity. The Snellen chart is one of the more commonly used (Fig. 1-1.) The chart is usually placed 20 feet from the patient. Under difficult technical circumstances, the chart could be placed 15 feet from the patient. The chart should be illuminated. Approximately 100-foot candles provide adequate illumination.

Acuity is recorded as a fraction. The numerator represents the distance to the chart and the denominator represents the distance at which a normal eye can read the line. Therefore, 20/200 indicates that the patient is 20 feet away and can read the line that a normal eye can read at 200 feet. Preschool children or illiterates should be tested with an illiterate "E" chart (Fig. 1-2). For this test, the patient is taught to point his finger in the direction of the "E" bars.

Visual acuity is examined one eye at a time. The other eye should be occluded. Pressure on the occluded eye should be avoided. The patient is asked to read with one eye as far down the chart as possible. This is recorded and the same procedure is repeated for the other eye.

If the patient wears glasses for distance vision, the test is repeated with glasses. The result should be recorded as "corrected visual acuity." The result without glasses is recorded as "uncorrected visual acuity."

A visual acuity less than the largest letter on the chart is recorded as finger counting (F. C.) at a certain distance, hand movements (H. M.), or light perception (L. P.). For example, the patient's visual acuity is finger counting at a distance of 5 feet. A poorer visual acuity is recorded as hand movements (H. M.) or light perception (L. P.). If an eye cannot perceive light, one should record "no light perception" (N. L. P.), rather than the confusing "BLIND" expression.

Measurement of near vision is relatively unimportant as a routine procedure in the emergency room. Under extremely poor technical conditions, the visual acuity chart for near can be used for persons under 35 years of age to determine visual acuity at 14 inches (Fig. 1-3). If the patient is 35 years or older, the visual acuity may be determined with his reading glasses.

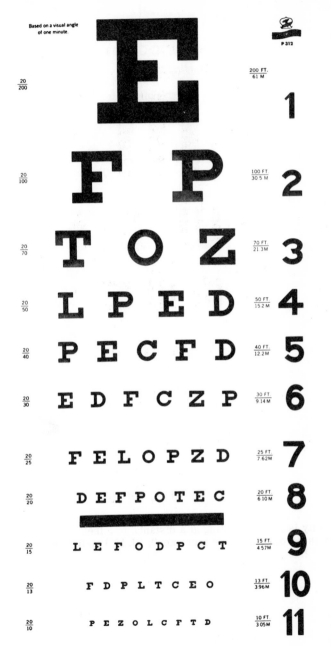

Based on a visual angle of one minute.

$\frac{20}{200}$	E	$\frac{200\ FT.}{61\ M}$ 1
$\frac{20}{100}$	F P	$\frac{100\ FT.}{30\ 5\ M}$ 2
$\frac{20}{70}$	T O Z	$\frac{70\ FT.}{21\ 3\ M}$ 3
$\frac{20}{50}$	L P E D	$\frac{50\ FT.}{15\ 2\ M}$ 4
$\frac{20}{40}$	P E C F D	$\frac{40\ FT.}{12\ 2\ M}$ 5
$\frac{20}{30}$	E D F C Z P	$\frac{30\ FT.}{9\ 14\ M}$ 6
$\frac{20}{25}$	F E L O P Z D	$\frac{25\ FT.}{7\ 62\ M}$ 7
$\frac{20}{20}$	D E F P O T E C	$\frac{20\ FT.}{6\ 10\ M}$ 8
$\frac{20}{15}$	L E F O D P C T	$\frac{15\ FT.}{4\ 57\ M}$ 9
$\frac{20}{13}$	F D P L T C E O	$\frac{13\ FT.}{3\ 96\ M}$ 10
$\frac{20}{10}$	P E Z O L C F T D	$\frac{10\ FT.}{3\ 05\ M}$ 11

Fig. 1-1. Visual acuity chart, based on a visual angle of one minute

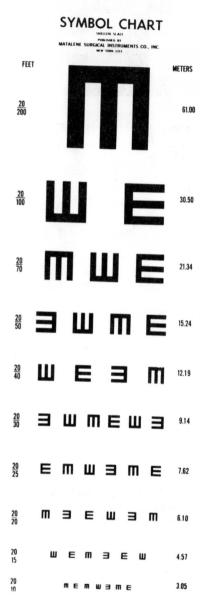

Fig. 1-2. Visual acuity chart for preschool children or illiterates

J. G. ROSENBAUM POCKET VISION SCREENER

					Point	Jaeger	distance equivalent
95							$\frac{20}{800}$
874							$\frac{20}{400}$
2843					26	16	$\frac{20}{200}$
6 3 8	⼛Ш⼛	X O O			14	10	$\frac{20}{100}$
8 7 4 5	⼛Ⅲ Ш	O X O			10	7	$\frac{20}{70}$
6 3 9 2 5	Ⅲ Ε ⼛	X O X			8	5	$\frac{20}{50}$
4 2 8 3 6 5	Ш Ε Ⅲ	O X O			6	3	$\frac{20}{40}$
3 7 4 2 5 8	⼛ Ш ⼛	x x O			5	2	$\frac{20}{30}$
9 3 7 8 2 6	Ш Ⅲ Ε	x O O			4	1	$\frac{20}{25}$
4 2 8 7 3 9	Ε Ш Ⅲ	O O x			3	1+	$\frac{20}{20}$

Card is held in good light 14 inches from eye.
Record vision for each eye separately with
and without glasses. Presbyopic patients
should read thru bifocal segment. Check
myopes with glasses only.

PUPIL GAUGE

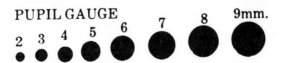

Fig. 1-3. J. G. Rosenbaum pocket vision screener

INSPECTION OF THE EXTERNAL OCULAR STRUCTURES

Inspection of the external ocular structures should include the lids (upper and lower), the lacrimal apparatus (gland, canaliculi, lacrimal sac, or dacryocyst), conjunctivas, corneas, scleras.

The examination is greatly facilitated by use of a well-focused source of light. The important objectives of lid examination are:

1. Detection of local disease or injury
2. Detection of local signs of systemic diseases
3. Inspection of the physiologic functions of the eyelids

Infection, retention cyst of the meibomian gland, traumatic wound of the eyelid, or infection of the dacryocyst, are only a few examples of local diseases to be detected by physical examination. Organic disease should be suspected in the case of lid edema, as this condition can be caused by systemic diseases of the heart or kidney organs. Abnormal closure or opening, dryness or tearing of the eye may lead the physician to different neurologic disturbances or abnormalities.

When there is history of an injury in which the coats of the eye may have been lacerated, great care should be taken to avoid pressure on the eyeball. The lids may be gently palpated by sliding a finger across the closed lid surface. The upper lid can be elevated by pressing upward over the brow (Fig. 1-4). The lower lid can be inspected by pulling the skin down with a finger over the bony maxilla (Fig. 1-5).

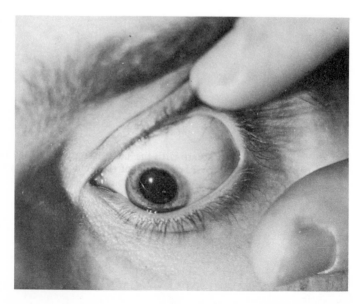

Fig. 1-4. The upper lid is elevated by pressing upward over the brow.

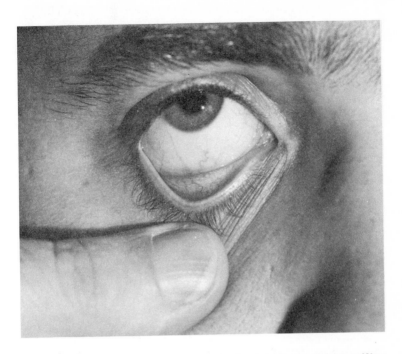

Fig. 1-5. The lower lid and conjunctival sac is inspected by pulling down the skin with a finger over the bony maxilla.

The upper eyelid is everted easily by grasping the lashes with one hand, pulling out and down, then pressing on the lid with a thin cotton applicator stick 1 cm above the edge of the lid margin, that is, at the superior border of the tarsal plate (Fig. 1-6). The patient is requested to look down during the entire procedure. Do not push the lids against the eyeball. In the presence of pain or lid spasm, it may be helpful to instill a few drops of sterile anesthetic solution in order to complete the examination properly. To restore the everted upper lid to its normal position, one should ask the patient to look up and simultaneously pull the lashes gently down.

The lacrimal apparatus starts with the lacrimal gland, which is situated at the superior temporal quadrant of the orbit. Part of it can be seen beneath the upper eyelid. Tears are carried from the gland to the lacrimal puncta, which is located at the nasal side of both lids. In the normal position these apertures touch the eye, the tears pass through the lacrimal canaliculi into the lacrimal sac, and from there via the nasal lacrimal duct to the nose.

Examination of the normal tear flow is especially important when the patient complains about dryness or excessive tearing. In addition to determining the patency of the lacrimal puncta and the canaliculi, attention should be given to the lacrimal sac, which can be obstructed and infected. This can be examined by applying pressure

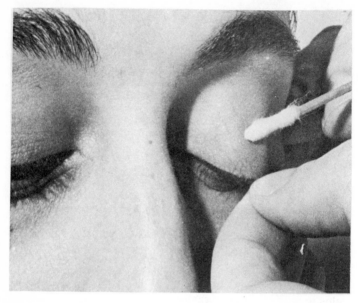

Fig. 1-6A. The upper eyelid eversion; grasp and pull down the lashes, pressing on the lid with a thin cotton applicator stick.

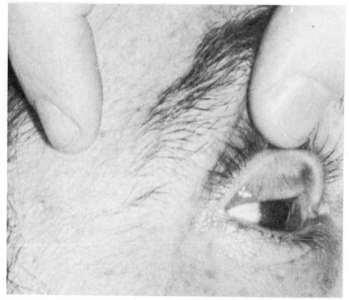

Fig. 1-6B. The everted eyelid

on the lacrimal sac for regurgitation of infected material. The pressure is directed inside the lower inner orbital rim, not on the nose.

EXAMINATION OF THE CONJUNCTIVA

The palpebral conjunctiva, which lines the posterior surface of the lid, is examined at the time of lid examination. The bulbar conjunctiva is easily examined by gentle separation of the lids and having the patient look up, down, left, and right. Normal conjunctiva is almost all white and transparent. Engorged vessel, secretion in different colors, can be symptoms of many eye diseases. In the case of a suspected conjunctival laceration, a drop of sterile fluorescein solution might help to detect the site of the injury.

CORNEA

The more sophisticated instruments to examine the cornea, such as the slit lamp, are not usually available in the emergency room. However, very often, important abnormalities of the cornea might be detected by simple external observation. Oblique illumination with a hand lamp is often sufficient to detect the pathology of important abnormalities such as abrasion or laceration of the cornea. Abrasions of the cornea are not always visible except when stained with fluorescein. A drop of sterile fluorescein solution or a piece of filter paper saturated with fluorescein, placed in the lower cul-de-sac, helps to locate corneal abrasion or surface debris or to differentiate abrasions from corneal opacities.

Corneal sensitivity is tested by gently touching a wisp of cotton to the center of the cornea. This examination should be performed before instilling any local anesthetic. The examiner should not touch the lashes or the lids and the patient should not see the approaching cotton since this causes blinking as much as the corneal sensitivity reflex. Comparison of the corneal reflexes of both eyes is the simplest and the best standard of reference. Loss of corneal sensitivity might be the sign of local eye disease (herpes keratitis) or neurologic abnormalities of the fifth cranial nerve.

POSITION OF THE EYES AND EYE MOVEMENTS

The size of the globe (microphthalmos = small eye, buphthalmos = large eye) and its position in the orbit should be noted. Tumor, inflammation, trauma, and thyroid disease may alter the normal position of the eyeball. When the eye is too much receded into the orbit the condition is called "enophthalmos." This could be one of the major signs of orbital floor fracture in case of a trauma to the orbit. "Exophthalmos" is the term used if the eye is displaced forward. Although abnormal displacements are recognizable by inspection, false impressions may be produced by unusual positions of the eyelid. (Widely open lids may simulate exophthalmos.) It may be necessary to take accurate measurements with an exophthalmometer.

MOVEMENTS OF THE EXTRAOCULAR MUSCLES

The eyes should be observed for movement together in all fields of gaze. By observing the reflection of light on the cornea one can examine the straightness of the eyes. For this purpose the easiest method is the use of a flashlight. This should be held directly in front of the patient at a distance of one foot. The patient is requested to look in the six cardinal positions of gaze, namely, left, right, up and right, up and left, down and right, down and left (Fig. 1-7).

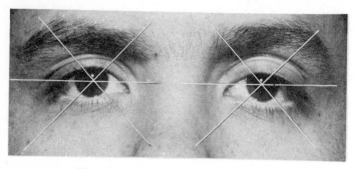

Fig. 1-7. Cardinal positions of gaze

Normally, the light reflection is symmetrical in both corneas. An asymmetric light reflex will betray a deviating eye. An ocular deviation could be caused by a paretic or paralytic extraocular muscle. Very often, early signs of a neurologic abnormality can be detected by careful examination of the extraocular muscles.

Nystagmus is an involuntary, rhythmically repeated oscillation of the eyes in any or all fields of gaze. Its importance and classification is discussed in the chapter on neuro-ophthalmologic emergencies.

PUPILS

The pupils should be inspected for:

1. Equality
2. Size
3. Shape
4. Reaction to stimulation (light reflex, accommodation reflex, consensual light response)

Inquiry should be made as to the use of any drug with mydriactic or miotic effect. Never use eyedrops to dilate the pupil prior to the examination of the pupil. Normal pupils are equal in size. Unequal pupils are called "anisocoria." Unequal pupils may suggest previous eye disease or neurologic disorder. The term "miosis" is used when pupils are smaller than 4 mm in diameter. This can be observed in case of an inflammation in the anterior segment of the eye. Morphine causes miosis. Physiologically, the pupil is miotic in sleep. The term "mydriasis" is used for enlarged pupils, that is, larger than 7 mm. The pupil is large in cases of ocular injury, systemic poisoning, and many neurologic diseases of the midbrain.

Generally, the shape of the pupil is round. Irregular pupils are almost always pathologic. The shape can be affected by congenital abnormalities or by other diseases such as iritis, syphilis, or trauma.

Examination for reaction to light is best performed in a semi-dark room. The light should be brought from the side. The pupil contracts to direct light. Constriction of the pupil of the other eye is called "consensual pupil reaction" to light. The reaction to accommodation is tested by holding one finger or a pencil a few inches in front of the eye being tested. The patient is requested to look at the pencil and at the far wall directly beyond the pencil. The pupil constricts when looking at the near object and dilates when looking at the far object. In general, if the pupil reacts to light, it reacts to accommodation as well. Argyl-Robertson pupil is a pathologic condition due to central nervous system syphilis in which there is a failure of direct and consensual light response, but there is a normal reaction to accommodation. Adie's pupil, or tonic pupil, responds to stimulation but very, very slowly.

MEASUREMENT OF INTRAOCULAR PRESSURE

The normal intraocular pressure is between 14-20 mm Hg. The more common procedures used to determine intraocular pressure are:

1. Finger tension
2. Measurement by Schiotz tonometer
3. Measurement by applanation tonometer

The simplest estimate of intraocular pressure is done by indenting the eye with the fingers (Fig. 1-8). The determination of intraocular pressure by finger is good only for gross evaluation. It is recommended that this type of examination is not done by the physician who is not familiar with the procedure since it can cause serious complications in the case of a lacerated eyeball.

Measuring the intraocular pressure with a Schiotz tonometer is strongly recommended (Fig. 1-9). This should be part of the general physical examination by the emergency room physician and the ophthalmologist as well. Tonometry by an instrument is contraindicated in the presence of an eye infection or in the case of an obvious perforation of the globe.

The procedure is as follows: An anesthetic solution is instilled in each eye. The patient lies on his back with his shirt collar open. All pressure in the neck should be relieved. The patient is requested to

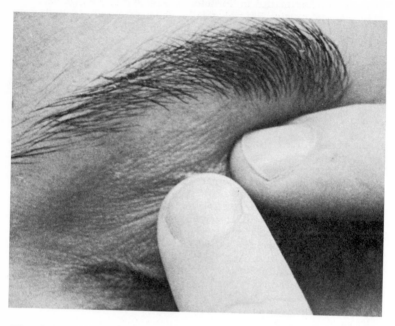

Fig. 1-8. Determination of intraocular pressure by finger technique

look at a spot on the ceiling with both eyes. The tonometer is placed in the middle of the corneal surface of each eye. The scale reading is taken from the tonometer. A special chart converts the scale reading to mm Hg. Tonometry by a Schiotz tonometer is accurate for clinical purposes in the emergency room and is adequate for primary diagnosis. To prevent spread of any ocular infection, the tonometer should be cleaned before and after each use.

The applanation tonometer is the more accurate method to measure intraocular pressure. This instrument is mounted on a slit lamp (Fig. 1-10). Applanation tonometry measures the force required to flatten the cornea. This technique is more accurate than tonometry by a Schiotz tonometer. In general, this is not available to the emergency room physician, and its use requires knowledge of perfect handling of the instrument and the slit lamp as well. Therefore, this method of measuring the intraocular pressure is more for the ophthalmologist rather than the general practitioner.

VISUAL FIELDS

Any complete eye examination includes the visual fields. Many conditions are associated with loss of visual field. Visual fields can be examined by:

1. Confrontation
2. Perimeter
3. Tangent screen

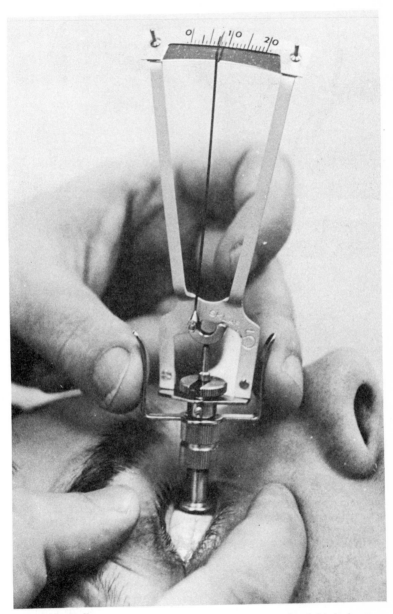

Fig. 1-9. Measurement of intraocular pressure by Schiotz tonometer

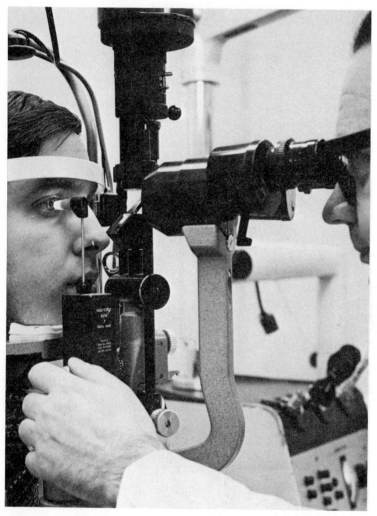

Fig. 1-10. Measurement of intraocular pressure by applanation
tonometer

CONFRONTATION

In general, special instruments for careful study are not available in the emergency room; however, the simple confrontation test should be used to examine the visual fields. This is a relatively rough test but gross visual field defects may be detected. The technique is as follows: The patient and the physician face each other at a distance of two feet. With one eye covered, the patient looks straight ahead at a specific fixation point (the physician's eye). A small object such as a pen or a pencil can be used as the target. The target is placed beyond the limits of the field of vision and advanced slowly forward. The patient is instructed to respond as soon as he sees the target. This is repeated at 8 to 10 equally spaced meridians through 360° (Fig. 1-11). The visual field is considered normal if the patient sees the target 90° temporally, 50° nasally, 50° upward, and 65° downward. The test is performed for each eye separately. Alterations in visual fields may be the result of ocular disease such as chorioretinitis or glaucoma, or neurologic disorders such as intracranial tumor or hemorrhage.

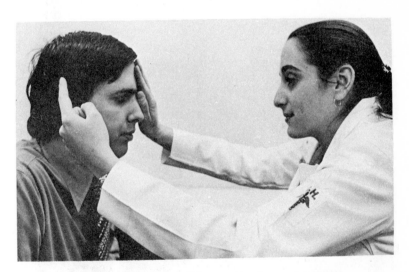

Fig. 1-11. Visual field examination by confrontation.

PERIMETER

For accurate examination of the peripheral visual field a perimeter is necessary (Fig. 1-12). Peripheral field examination by perimeter is indicated when the physician detects constriction of the peripheral field by confrontation or he suspects ocular or neurologic disorder

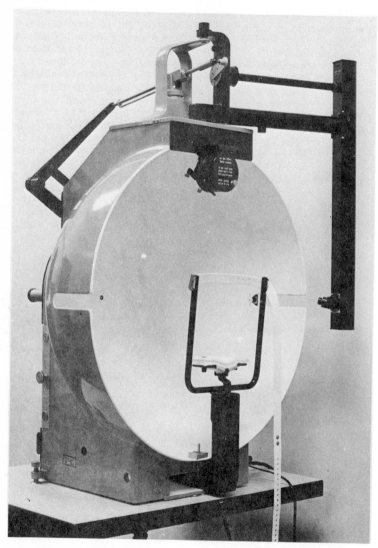

Fig. 1-12. The Goldmann perimeter

which may cause peripheral field defect. It must be carefully explained to the patient, before examination, that accurate responses are important. The patient is seated at the instrument with one eye covered. The patient's chin is placed on the chin rest. The patient is asked to fixate on the central spot of the perimeter. The eye is now 33 cm from the test target in any direction. The test target, in the case of the Goldmann perimeter, is a light which is brought in from the side. The patient is asked to signal immediately when he sees the target. As in the case of confrontation, 8 to 10 equally spaced meridians are examined through 360°. Each eye is tested separately. If a smaller target is used for examination, the possibility of detecting a scotoma in the visual field is greater.

TANGENT SCREEN

Central visual fields are examined with a tangent screen. Many physicians feel that this diagnostic test of visual fields is the most important and accurate. The patient is seated one or two meters from the tangent screen. The examination is performed as in the case of perimetry, which is described above (Fig. 1-13). One should not forget that examinations of the visual fields are subjective tests and vary markedly with fatigue, lack of concentration, and lack of cooperation with the examiner.

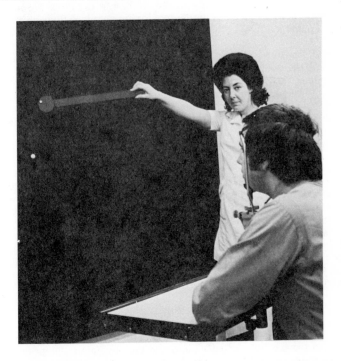

Fig. 1-13. Visual field examination by tangent screen. The patient's head is on the chin rest opposite to the center of the screen.

FUNDUSCOPY

One of the more important parts of the eye examination is the examination of the posterior segment. This is done with an ophthalmoscope. There are three types of instruments which can be used to examine the posterior segment. They are as follows:

1. Direct ophthalmoscope
2. Indirect ophthalmoscope
3. Contact glass with three mirrors

The last two require special knowledge and experience and, therefore, their use is recommended only to the trained ophthalmologist.

The examination is more easily accomplished through a dilated pupil. One or two drops of Mydriacyl 1% solution (tropicamid), or any other mydriatic eye drop, is used to dilate the pupil within a few minutes and greatly simplifies the examination.

In the young patient, the danger of the mydriatic precipitating an attack of acute angle-closure glaucoma is negligible. In the older patient it is advisable to estimate the depth of the anterior chamber either with the direct ophthalmoscope or by means of oblique illumination. If the anterior chambers are shallow it is better not to dilate the pupils but rather examine the posterior segment through the undilated pupil.

The illumination in the room should be decreased. The examination requires the cooperation of the patient in that he must hold his eyes still; also, the patient must follow the instructions of the examiner concerning eye movements in different directions.

These rules should be observed regardless of the type of ophthalmoscope used for the examination.

DIRECT OPHTHALMOSCOPY

There are many types of direct ophthalmoscopes. Source of illumination is provided either by batteries or from a wall outlet. The two main advantages of direct ophthalmoscopy are (a) easy handling, and (b) magnification of the picture (about 14 times).

The ophthalmoscope is held in the physician's right hand and in front of his right eye, sitting or standing at the right side of the patient when examining the patient's right eye (Fig. 1-14). The left hand and the left eye are used from the left side to examine the left eye.

PART "A" OF THE FUNDUS EXAMINATION

The lens wheel is rotated to the +10 diopter lens. The light beam is directed toward the patient's pupil and the physician brings the instrument close to the eye. First the reflex of the fundus is seen. If the eye ground is normal the reflex is red. The examiner then

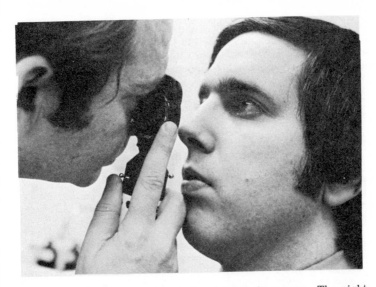

Fig. 1-14. Funduscopy using a direct ophthalmoscope. The right hand and the right eye is used from the right side to examine the right fundus.

gradually reduces the strength of the plus lens. The focus of observation gradually progresses through the vitreous to the retina. If the lens is cataractous or the vitreous is hazy, the red reflex cannot be seen. Massive vitreous hemorrhage can cause a black fundus reflex.

PART "B" OF THE FUNDUS EXAMINATION

If the fundus is visible, the optic disc should be examined first (Fig. 1-15). The disc can be found easily if the light is directed into the eye from a slightly temporal direction to the straight-ahead gaze of the patient.

First, the color of the disc is noted. The hyperemic disc is pink, while the atrophic disc has a grayish color. The border of the disc should be carefully examined. The normal disc has a well-defined border. Occasionally, the border of the normal disc can be blurred. This condition, called pseudopapilledema, is a rare variation of normal. A disc with a blurred border usually indicates the presence of disease. In the case of elevated intracranial pressure, the condition is called papilledema; in the case of an inflammatory process of the nerve head, papillitis (Fig. 1-16).

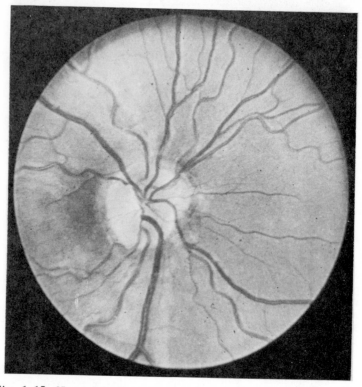

Fig. 1-15. Normal fundus appearance, the disc with the major vessels

PART "C" OF THE FUNDUS EXAMINATION

The next step in the fundus examination is inspection of the vessels. The route of each main artery should be followed from the disc to the periphery, and that of each main vein from the periphery back to the disc. Narrow arteries, dilated veins, A-V compressions, hemorrhages, and exudates around the vessels should be noted. Round hemorrhages may occur in the patient with diabetes mellitus. Flame-shaped hemorrhages is a common finding in the patient with high blood pressure.

PART "D" OF THE FUNDUS EXAMINATION

The macular area is examined as the fourth part of the fundus examination. The easiest way is to ask the patient to look into the light of

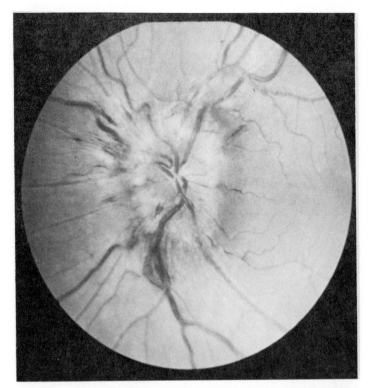

Fig. 1-16. Optic disc showing signs of papilledema: blurred disc margin, dilated veins and hemorrhages around the disc.

the ophthalmoscope. Normally, a red reflex of the avascular macular area is seen. In case of edema or degeneration of the retina at the macular area, the macular reflex is absent or diminished.

PART "E" OF THE FUNDUS EXAMINATION

In the last part of the fundus examination an all-around search for pathology is performed by looking into the equatorial area and the periphery of the fundus. Fundus lesions should be located and measured. The size of a lesion is estimated by comparing it with the size of the optic disc. The size of the optic disc averages 1. 5 mm. The distance of the lesion from the disc or from the macula is recorded also. For example: The lesion is 1-disc diameter in size, is 4-disc diameters distant from the macula at the 11-o'clock position.

INDIRECT OPHTHALMOSCOPY

Indirect ophthalmoscopy is used mainly by the ophthalmologist (Fig. 1-17). In general, the emergency room physician is not trained to use this instrument. The advantages of this type of examination are: (a) the illumination is stronger than that of the direct ophthalmoscope. The light may pass through opacities of the vitreous and the fundus can be visualized; (b) the fundus picture appears in three dimensions. The main disadvantage of this method is that only the well-trained ophthalmologist can perform the fundus examination with the indirect ophthalmoscope. An additional disadvantage is that the observed image is smaller than that with the direct ophthalmoscope. The magnification of the fundus is only 3 or 4 times, whereas with the direct ophthalmoscope, it is 14 times.

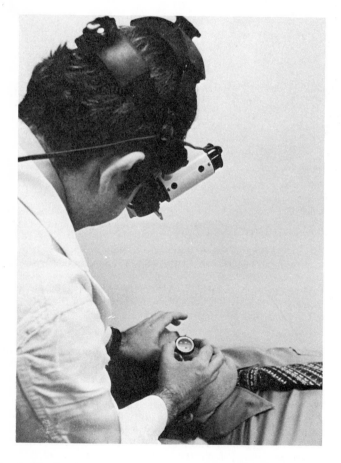

Fig. 1-17. Fundus examination by indirect ophthalmoscopy. The light source is on the head of the examiner. A 18 D lens is held in front of the eye of the patient.

CONTACT GLASS EXAMINATION

The contact glass examination is reserved for the ophthalmologist only (Fig. 1-18). Therefore, it is mentioned only briefly. The examination is performed with the aid of a slit lamp. A contact glass with three mirrors is placed on the cornea after instillation of a local anesthetic solution. This type of examination provides a highly magnified, well-illuminated, and three-dimensional picture of the fundus.

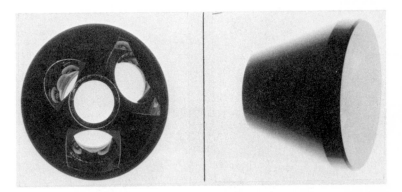

Fig. 1-18. Goldmann 3-mirror contact glass

III. SPECIAL EXAMINATIONS: The special examinations discussed in this section are not absolutely necessary to establish a diagnosis in the emergency room. However, they may provide considerable aid and can direct the ophthalmologist toward proper evaluation and treatment. In this chapter we will not mention all the sophisticated methods of eye examinations presently used in ophthalmology, but we will restrict the discussion to those methods which may actually be helpful in an emergency situation.

SLIT-LAMP EXAMINATION

The slit lamp is a binocular microscope with a strong source of light (Fig. 1-19). It provides a highly magnified and well-illuminated view of the area which might be involved in disease or trauma. The instrument is especially useful when one suspects a small foreign body or laceration of the cornea.

The patient places his chin on the chin rest and his forehead presses slightly against the plastic frame. The ophthalmologist examines the

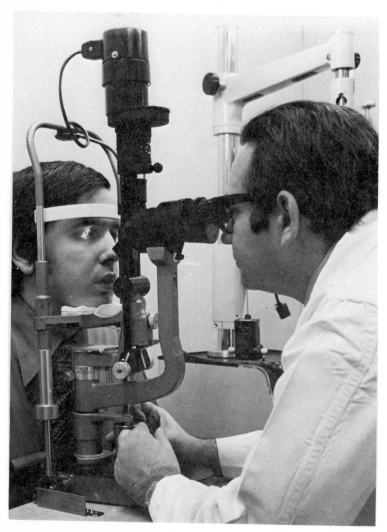

Fig. 1-19. Slit-lamp examination

eyes by moving the instrument into focus with a small handle situated on the table of the instrument. The lids and the anterior segment of the eye can be examined easily. If the pupil is dilated, the lens is checked for opacities or dislocation. To examine the posterior segment of the eye, special attachments are necessary. The slit lamp is used with the Hruby lens attachment or with a contact glass placed on the cornea.

EXOPHTHALMOMETRY

Although abnormal prominence or backward displacement of the eye is recognizable by inspection, proper measurements may be taken with the exophthalmometer (Fig. 1-20). With the exophthalmometer, one can measure the antero-posterior distance between the most anterior part of the cornea and the lateral orbital rim. The exophthalmometer is placed against the bony orbital margin on both sides and the bar reading is noted. This number is the distance in millimeters between the two bony orbital walls. The physician then views the corneas in the instrument's mirror. The corneas are simultaneously lined up with a scale in millimeters. The measurements are noted again. Both the bar reading and the protrusion of the eyes are recorded. Example: 98-19/18 means that the bar reading is 98 mm; right eye protrudes 19 mm; left eye, 18 mm. For successive comparative measurements, the bar reading of the same patient should always be the same. Normal range of protrusion of the eyes averages between 12-20 millimeters. Exophthalmic measurements are over 21 millimeters (Fig. 1-21). If there is no protrusion, both eyes should give equal or almost equal measurements.

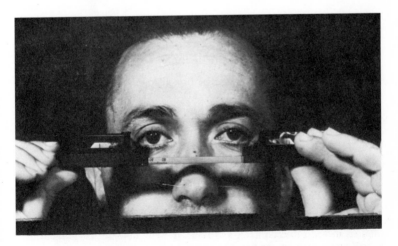

Fig. 1-20. Exophthalmometry. The exophthalmometer measures the antero-posterior distance between the most anterior part of the cornea and the bony lateral orbital rim.

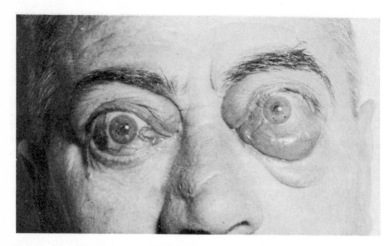

Fig. 1-21. Bilateral exophthalmos and chemosis. The right eye
protrudes 25 millimeters, the left eye protrudes 26
millimeters.

X-RAY

X-ray examination of the eye and orbit is discussed in a separate
chapter.

BACTERIOLOGIC EXAMINATION

Bacteriologic examinations are indicated in external infection with
secretion, or in suspected intraocular infection before starting any
treatment. The procedure is divided into two parts. First, the suspected area (corneal ulcer) is scraped with a sterile spatula or secretion material is removed from the lower cul-de-sac and smeared
on a glass slide. After this material is dried, the smear is stained
with one of the commonly available stains (Gram, Giemsa, KOH).
The smear is then studied under the microscope. Bacteria or hyphae
of fungus, eosinophils or other white cells can be identified in this
manner.

The second part of the examination consists of taking culture sam-
ples from the infected area and from the cul-de-sac for incubation
in different culture media. This part of the examination can be very
helpful if the initial treatment proved to be ineffective, and a change
in treatment is indicated, based on the findings of the cultures.

CHAPTER 2

SUDDEN LOSS OR DETERIORATION OF VISION

Sudden loss or deterioration of vision is an important ophthalmologic emergency. In most cases the deterioration of vision is painless and the patient is rarely aware of its seriousness. The emergency room physician must be alerted to this problem and diagnose the cause of deteriorated vision within a relatively short period of time. Early diagnosis and immediate treatment might restore useful vision in many cases. The patient's age, past history, general health, and a possible history of injury are all important factors which help the physician to establish the correct diagnosis. As an example, a young adult with a previous history of sudden loss of vision presents himself again in the emergency room because of deteriorated vision. Most likely the diagnosis will be recurrent optic neuritis. As an additional example, an elderly individual with general arteriosclerosis, complaining of markedly reduced vision which occurred recently, most likely will have vascular occlusion of the retina.

Sudden loss or serious deterioration of vision can be caused by the following:

1. Optic neuritis (retrobulbar neuritis, ischemic optic neuritis, temporal arteritis)
2. Hysteria
3. Vitreous hemorrhage
4. Vascular occlusions of the retina
5. Retinal detachment
6. Poisoning
7. Acute attack of glaucoma
8. Acute chorioretinitis at the macula
9. Retinal hemorrhage at the macula
10. Trauma

Optic neuritis and hysteria are described in detail in the chapter on neuro-ophthalmologic emergencies. Glaucoma and trauma will be discussed in their corresponding chapters.

VITREOUS HEMORRHAGE

Hemorrhage into the vitreous body is a serious disorder. It can be related to systemic disease or it can be caused by a disease of the eye. Trauma also is an important cause of vitreous hemorrhage. Main causes of vitreous hemorrhage include:

1. Hemopoetic disease
2. Increased arterial pressure
3. Increased venous pressure
4. Inflamed vessels
5. Arteriovenous malformation

6. Neovascularization of the retina
7. Retinal tears
8. Vitreoretinal traction
9. Degenerative disease of the choroid
10. Intraocular surgery
11. Intraocular tumor
12. Trauma

Diabetes mellitus and hypertension are two of the more frequent underlying causes of vitreous hemorrhage caused by systemic disease. Retinal tears, central retinal vein occlusion, and tumor are the more common eye diseases causing massive vitreous hemorrhage. Hemorrhage due to hemopoetic disorder is less frequent. This group includes leukemia, thrombocytopenia, anemia, macroglobulinemia, and drug-induced hemorrhages caused, for example, by anticoagulant overdose or hemolytic reaction to certain therapeutic agents.

Hemorrhage may originate in the retinal vessels, the choroid, or the ciliary body. One or both eyes can be affected, sometimes both eyes are involved at the same time.

Experimental investigations show that the blood in the vitreous body clots rapidly, forming a red mass with sharp borders. This occurs mainly because of the latticework of vitreous collagen fibers, with large hyaluronic acid molecules in the interspaces that retard the diffusion of red cells. Additional factors causing rapidly clotting blood is a thromboplastin-like substance in the vitreous, analogous to activated factor X which accelerates clotting.

In the retrovitreal space, the blood remains fluid.

The clot in the vitreous starts to break down within a few days. Erythrocyte debris are removed by leukocytes and plasma cells. The chemical factor which causes these cells to enter the vitreous is not known. Strong experimental and clinical evidence indicates that in man the erythrocyte debris drain mainly anteriorly through the trabecular meshwork of the anterior chamber. Debris of blood may elicit inflammatory response in the iris. Also, they are toxic to the endothelial cells of the trabecular meshwork, the epithelium of the ciliary body, the retinal pigment epithelium, and the sensory retina.

It is still not well known whether the iron is the toxic agent, whether the hemoglobin itself is responsible directly for toxic changes in the eye, or hemosiderin causes degeneration of the ocular tissues.

SIGNS AND SYMPTOMS: There is a sudden loss or deterioration of vision of the affected eye. The anterior segment rarely shows any abnormality except dilatation of the pupil. The normal red reflex of the fundus is diminished or absent. The fundus reflex is black rather than red. Details of the retina cannot be seen because of the cloudy media.

TREATMENT: Unfortunately, there is no effective therapy for vitreous hemorrhage. Bed rest, with the head elevated, helps the blood to gravitate to the bottom of the vitreous cavity.

Vitreous hemorrhage may be treated with enzymes such as strepto-kinase-streptodornase (Varidase), collagenase, or fibrinolysin. The rationale behind treatment with streptokinase-streptodornase is that enzymes liquefy the vitreous gel permitting easier diffusion and settling of blood to the bottom of the eye. Fibrinolysin is believed to accelerate lysis of blood clot. There is no definite proof that enzy-matic treatment is helpful in vitreous hemorrhage and, therefore, few ophthalmologists use enzymes in the treatment of such cases.

The use of systemic steroids also is controversial. Experimental studies indicated that ACTH delays resorbtion of blood from the vi-treous. On the other hand, a few clinical surveys report that the use of systemic steroids rapidly clears the vitreous.

PROGNOSIS AND LATE COMPLICATIONS OF VITREOUS HEMOR-RHAGE: Vitreous hemorrhage may clear within a few days or weeks; however, in certain cases blood remains in the vitreous for months. The prognosis with regard to visual acuity seems to correlate with the size of the hemorrhage and is worsened by recurrent episodes.

Vitreous hemorrhage can cause hemolytic glaucoma by damaging the trabecular meshwork and blocking the aqueous outflow. Neovas-cular hemorrhagic glaucoma also can result from vitreous hemor-rhage. It is not yet clear if this type of glaucoma is directly caused by vitreous hemorrhage or if it is due to other conditions causing the vitreous hemorrhage. Siderotic glaucoma is due to iron-induced chronic degenerative changes in the trabecular meshwork.

Other late complications include connective tissue proliferation into the vitreous body. This proliferative tissue may cause retinal de-tachment or additional hemorrhage by pulling on the retina.

Because of the almost complete failure of drug therapy, mechanical means of removing the opaque vitreous from the eye, that is, partial vitrectomy, may be considered in certain cases a few months after hemorrhage. There are many hazards in vitreous surgery; however, in selective cases it might be worthwhile to remove the blood or the fibrotic proliferative tissue before they cause irreversible damage to the vitreous and the retina.

Serious impairment or complete loss of vision is not an unusual end result of massive vitreous hemorrhage.

RETINAL VASCULAR OCCLUSION

The vascular occlusion of the retina can be divided into two groups:

1. Arterial occlusion
2. Venous occlusion

In either group, occlusions may occur in the branch only or in the central vessel.

1. RETINAL ARTERY OCCLUSION

The etiology of occlusion of a retinal artery is usually not immediately apparent. Artheromatosis of the vessel is the most common cause among older people. Emboli in the presence of heart disease such as auricular fibrillation is another relatively common etiologic factor (Fig. 2-1). However, occlusion of retinal artery may occur even in the absence of arteriosclerosis, heart disease, or any other detectable systemic or local disease. The cause of occlusion in the healthy young adult is unknown. Whether the vascular obstruction is due to a spastic closure of the vessel in these cases is still unknown. Spastic closure of arteries have been noted among females below middle age. On rare occasions an angiospasm may be due to toxins - endogenous such as pregnancy or exogenous such as lead or quinine. Retinal artery occlusion caused by cranial arteritis, polyarteritis, pulseless disease, carotid occlusion, essential hypotension, sudden drop in blood pressure, following ocular or orbital surgery, orbital granuloma, orbital infection, sickle cell disease, parasite, or trauma is much more rare. Occlusion of the retinal artery is not a common disease. Early diagnosis and immediate treatment might be sight-saving.

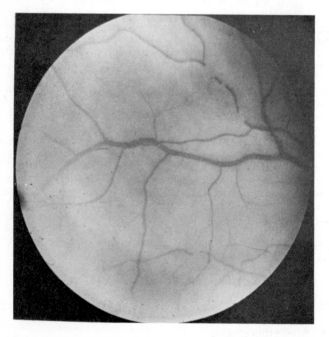

Fig. 2-1. Multiple emboli in the upper temporal retinal artery. Medical investigation proved that the emboli originated from an eroded atheromatous plaque in the common carotid artery.

When the occlusion is confined to a branch vessel, the superior temporal branch vessel is involved most frequently.

In cases where histologic examination could be performed, edema of
the nerve fibers layer and of the ganglion cells layer have been
found. The outer part, including the neuroepithelium, and the outer
molecular layer remain intact since they are supplied by choriocapillaries. If obstruction has been discovered histologically, the
obstruction occurs usually at the lamina cribosa, the intraneural
segment of the artery, or its exit from the nerve.

SIGNS AND SYMPTOMS: There is a sudden painless deterioration
of vision of the affected eye. The visual acuity can be reduced to
light perception or complete blindness. The pupil is wide and does
not react to a direct light stimulus. On fundus examination, the disc
is pale and the veins appear dark. The arterioles are narrowed and
less frequently show sludging. There is marked edema of the retina
corresponding to the occluded artery. If the central retinal artery
is occluded, the whole posterior pole is edematous and, except for
the fovea, appears whitish (Fig. 2-2). The foveal area transmits its
normal red choroidal color because at the fovea the retina is thin
and the choroidal blood supply shows through. This is known as the
"cherry red" spot, a sign of occlusion of the central retinal artery.

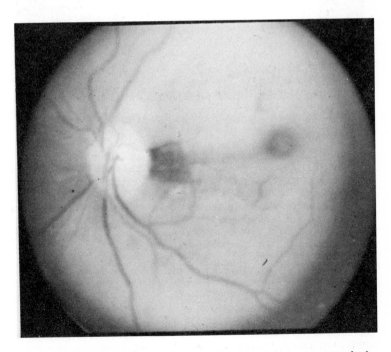

Fig. 2-2. Retinal artery occlusion. The foveal area appears dark
when compared to the surrounding retina, which is pale
and edematous.

In branch occlusion, the pallor of the fundus is confined to the area supplied by the affected artery (Fig. 2-3).

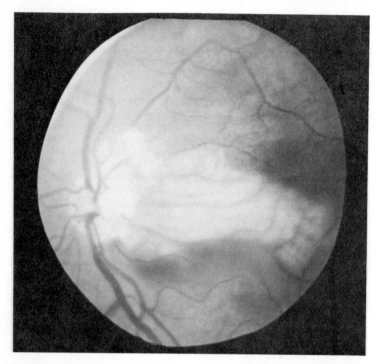

Fig. 2-3. Branch occlusion of the retinal artery. The pallor is confined to the area served by the affected artery.

TREATMENT: For the most part, treatment of this condition is sometimes ineffective. Ophthalmologists have tried different therapeutic procedures. Surgery such as iridectomy or paracentesis is now used less often. Medical therapy may include anticoagulant treatment, thrombolytic enzymes with or without anticoagulant therapy, and vasodilators alone or in combination with anticoagulants. Recently, low molecular weight dextran was added to the pharmacologic armoury to treat occlusion of retinal artery.

If treatment of an arterial occlusion is delayed the visual results will be poor. It is not known how long the retina can tolerate any loss or diminution of its blood supply. However, it is evident from clinical experience that if treatment is delayed for more than 12 hours, and significant edema of the retina is present, successful response to any kind of therapy is unlikely. Therefore, quick diagnosis and immediate treatment is imperative.

EMERGENCY TREATMENTS: A recently published complex therapy provides relatively good results and is recommended herein. After establishment of the diagnosis a short general medical examination should be performed to exclude major medical contraindication to the contemplated treatment, which is the following:

1. Retrobulbar injection of 2 ml of 2% xylocaine hydrochloride and 200 mg acetylcholine. (In severe heart conditions and asthma it is better to avoid the administration of acetylcholine to prevent complication from the administration of this drug itself).

2. The above-mentioned is followed by intravenous administration of low molecular weight dextran (Rheomacrodex, Gentran 40) and papaverine hydrochloride. During the first 24 hours of treatment 1500 ml of a 10% solution of low molecular weight dextran with 300 mg of papaverine hydrochloride are infused. On each of the following four days the patient is given intravenously 500 ml of dextran with 100 mg of papaverine hydrochloride of which additional intravenous injections (50 mg each) are administered every 6-8 hours to bring the total daily dose to 200 mg.

Low molecular weight dextran, on the other hand, was shown to be effective when arterial obstruction is present or the capillary flow is impaired. Low molecular weight dextran reduces the whole blood viscosity and has a specific disaggregating effect on human erythrocytes. It has been shown that low molecular weight dextran inhibits thrombus formation and propagation, thus interfering with the first stage of thrombus formation.

During the patient's stay in the hospital medical examinations and laboratory tests should be performed in an attempt to determine the presence of disease which possibly could cause an arterial occlusion. Visual acuity, visual field, and ophthalmoscopy examinations should be performed daily to detect any improvement in or worsening of the condition of the affected eye.

Another emergency treatment used by many ophthalmologists consists of CO_2 inhalation. It is believed that inhaling CO_2 of high concentration (5%) causes vasodilatation of the retinal vessels. Inhalations should be repeated at regular intervals.

Retrobulbar injection of tolazoline hydrochloride (Priscoline) in amounts of 25 mg is used in a few medical centers.

Inhalation of amyl nitrite and the oral administration of other nitrites and nicotinic acid have little therapeutic effect on the retinal vessels and, therefore, their use as an emergency treatment is of little value in retinal artery occlusion.

Anticoagulant treatment is still widely used. This was the treatment of choice for many years. However, based on the clinical experience of many ophthalmologists, significant improvement has been achieved only rarely, if at all, with this kind of treatment and, therefore, now it is less recommended. It is especially not recommended for an elderly person or a patient with a history of bleeding tendency.

PROGNOSIS: The retina can survive hypoxia and reduced blood supply for longer periods of time than the brain. The prognosis is not hopeless. Good results are reported if the treatment is instituted within a few hours after the occlusion occurs.

There is no known way to predict the end result of a branch or central retinal artery occlusion. Fortunately, it is rare that an arterial occlusion will occur in both eyes simultaneously.

2. OCCLUSION OF THE CENTRAL RETINAL VEIN
OCCLUSION OF A BRANCH RETINAL VEIN

Thrombosis of the central retinal vein is a rare but serious condition. Thrombosis usually occurs at the level of the lamina cribosa of the optic nerve. In this area the artery and the vein are very close to each other, enclosed within the same adventitial tissue sheath. Sclerotic changes in the artery compress the lumen of the vein. In addition, artheromatous changes in the artery slows down the circulation to the retina - an important factor for thrombus formation within the sclerosed vein already suffering from compression. This pathogenesis is well understood in the elderly or the middle-aged patient who often suffers from hypertension or general arteriosclerosis. Central vein occlusion may occur in a hematologic abnormality such as polycythemia, leukemia, or macroglobulinemia. In addition to these etiologic factors, some cases of vein occlusions are of uncertain etiology and pathogenesis, especially among young healthy adults. Vein occlusion may be due also to inflammation-phlebitis, parasitic obstruction, pressure on the vein from tumor, increased orbital and intraocular pressure and sudden reduction of systemic blood pressure.

If the obstruction affects only one division of the central retinal vein, the condition is called branch occlusion.

When branch occlusion is present, the pathology is confined to the sector of the occluded vein. The etiologic factors and pathogenesis of branch occlusion are probably the same as those of central retinal vein occlusion.

SIGNS AND SYMPTOMS: Sudden or gradual but severe deterioration of visual acuity occurs in central vein occlusion. Visual acuity may be reduced to hand movements or light perception only. The visual acuity change is less severe in branch occlusion. The visual field defect corresponds to the retina damaged by the occlusion. The deterioration of vision is painless in most cases.

The anterior segment of the eye shows little involvement. Occasionally, the vessels in the iris are dilated and engorged. The ophthalmoscopic picture of the central retinal vein is typical. The optic disc is deep red and its border is blurred because of swelling.

Multiple hemorrhages are seen all around the optic disc and the posterior pole. The size and shape of the hemorrhages are variable. The hemorrhages may be small or large, flame-shaped or round. They may be superficial or deep. The arteries are narrow. The veins are engorged and their color is much darker than in the normal fundus. White patchy exudates may be seen all around. Cotton wool patches, when present, are more frequent around the optic disc (Fig. 2-4).

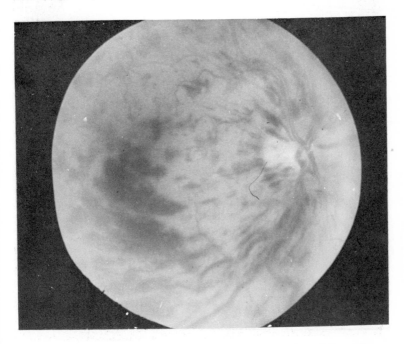

Fig. 2-4. Central retinal vein occlusion. The border of the optic disc is hardly seen. Multiple hemorrhages of different size and shape are seen all around the posterior pole. The veins are considerably engorged.

The ophthalmoscopic appearance of the branch occlusion is much less dramatic. The optic disc is rarely involved. Hemorrhages, exudates, and vascular changes can be seen all around the occluded vein. As in the case of central retinal vein occlusion, the size and shape of the hemorrhages and exudates are variable (Fig. 2-5).

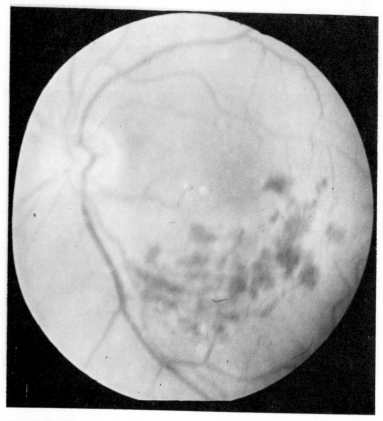

Fig. 2-5. Branch occlusion of the central retinal vein. Hemorrhages are seen along the occluded vessel.

DIFFERENTIAL DIAGNOSIS: The central vein occlusion is a unilateral disease. Ophthalmoscopic appearance is similar to that of papilledema. However, in papilledema usually both eyes are involved and the vision is good, while in vein occlusion the visual acuity is reduced.

The same is true in a case of severe hypertension; both eyes are involved almost equally and the vision is relatively good. The pathologic fundus signs are bilateral also in other systemic diseases such as diabetes or hemorrhagic disorders.

When branch vein occlusion is diagnosed, vasculitis must be considered in the differential diagnosis.

TREATMENT: The conventional treatment is short-term or long-term anticoagulant therapy. Heparin reduces immediately the co-agulability of the blood. Coumarin or coumadrin reduces the pro-thrombin in the blood and in this way interferes with normal coagu-lation and thrombus formation. Anticoagulant therapy is onerous, not without risk, and very often disappointing. The use of urokinase 150, 000 units administered over a period of three days is another treatment of doubtful value.

Vasodilators such as long-acting papaverine or cyclandelate (Cyclo-spasmol) may be of some help. The rationale of this treatment is that diminished arterial flow to the retinal circulation causes stasis of the blood in the veins. Therefore, vasodilator drugs provide bet-ter arterial blood flow, reduce congestion and, therefore, the pos-sibility of vein occlusion. Recently, the combination of low molecu-lar weight dextran and vasodilators has been used to treat venous occlusion. The results are promising. This treatment is the same as that for arterial occlusion. It has been described previously in full detail under "treatment of central retinal artery occlusion."

PROGNOSIS: Useful vision may be restored in 10%-20% of patients. In most cases, the final visual acuity is between 20/200 and 20/400. New vessel formation may be seen in the fundus, most commonly on the optic disc. Secondary glaucoma is a complication of central vein occlusion. It is infrequent in branch occlusion.

RETINAL DETACHMENT

Detachment of the retina may cause gradual or sudden deterioration of vision. The condition is not a true detachment of the retina from the choroid. The so-called "detachment" is actually a separation of the two primitive layers of the retina. The hexagon pigment layer remains attached to Bruch's membrane and the rest of the choroid, and only the sensory retina is detached. "Subretinal fluid" accumu-lates between the pigment epithelium layer and the sensory retina. If the retina is detached only at the periphery, the visual acuity is not impaired seriously. However, if the detachment extends into the macular area the vision is markedly deteriorated. Thus, retinal detachment is a true emergency if the macula is threatened.

Retinal detachment can be classified as primary or secondary, rhegmatogenous or non-rhegmatogenous. Duke-Elder classifies retinal detachments as follows:

A. Exudative detachments
B. Traction detachments
C. Perforated detachments (rhegmatogenous)

The role of trauma in the etiology of retinal detachment is generally an accessory to the main pathogenic factors which are changes in the vitreous, in the retina, and probably in the choroid. A severe trauma without the previously mentioned pathogenic factors also may cause retinal detachment (see retinal detachment in the chapter on trauma). However, in the case of the "usual retinal detachment," the trauma is only a triggering factor. The incidence of retinal detachment varies from country to country. The incidence is affected by sex, age, myopia, heredity, race, and aphakia. In the United States and in Europe the average annual incidence is estimated between 8 to 18 per 100,000 people. Strong evidence indicates that Negroes are affected less than Caucasians. Retinal detachment may occur in both eyes in about 25% of cases.

SIGNS AND SYMPTOMS: The patient may complain of cloudy, smoky vision, occasional lightning flashes or sparks. Later, the patient complains of a shadow or curtain which obscures a portion of the visual field. If the detachment does not involve the macula the visual acuity may remain normal. A severe loss in central vision occurs when the macula area is detached. Often, the patient does not consider seriously the signs of peripheral retinal detachment, namely, seeing a shadow, and comes to the emergency room because of sudden deterioration of vision when detachment of the macula occurs. The visual acuity may be reduced to finger counting. At first, the visual field defect is relative. The color vision defect is of the tritanopic type. In most cases the intraocular pressure remains normal or slightly below normal. The detached retina looks grey, occasionally with white folds in it. Also, the detached retina may have a globular bullous appearance (Fig. 2-6). The folds of the retina may resemble hills and valleys. In a rhegmatogenous detachment, retinal holes or tears should be present. Holes may appear horseshoe-shaped or round. In most cases the holes occur at the equatorial area or peripheral to it. It is not always easy to find the hole or holes in a case of retinal detachment. The young physician with limited experience will not detect them easily.

DIFFERENTIAL DIAGNOSIS: Primary retinal detachment must be differentiated from the so-called secondary retinal detachment such as that due to primary or metastatic tumor of the choroid. Fluorescein fundus angiography is the most reliable diagnostic test to rule out mitotic lesion and to differentiate between rhegmatogenous retinal detachment and retinal detachment caused by a tumor. Ultrasound and P_{32} also are very useful laboratory examinations and have important diagnostic value in this respect. Other types of secondary detachment, such as retinal detachment in toxemia of pregnancy or in kidney disease, is almost always bilateral and involves the lower half of the retina. The severity of general condition of the patient and the known systemic diseases also are helpful to make the correct diagnosis. If the emergency room physician is not sure of the diagnosis there is always sufficient time to consult an experienced ophthalmologist.

TREATMENT: Whenever a primary retinal detachment is diagnosed, immediate admission to the hospital is necessary. Bed rest is essential. Repeated ophthalmoscopic examinations should be performed in order to determine the nature of the detachment and the location of retinal tears and holes.

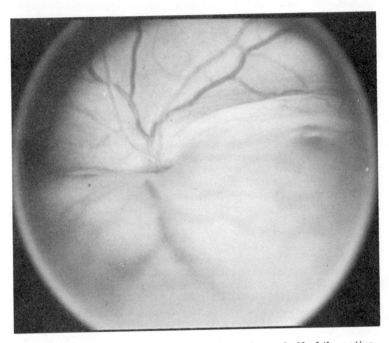

Fig. 2-6. Bullous retinal detachment. The lower half of the retina is detached.

If the macula area is detached, surgical intervention is required as soon as possible. The longer the macula remains detached, the less likely is the possibility to regain good vision after surgery. Loss of central vision can be permanent even after the retina has been successfully reattached.

Reattachment of retina can be accomplished only by surgery. Spontaneous reattachment is rare. Without surgery the retinal detachment becomes total, resulting in permanent blindness within one-half to two years.

The primary goal of surgery is to seal the retinal holes causing choroidal inflammation and exudates. The holes are sealed either by diathermy or cryosurgery through the area of the sclera corresponding to the retinal defects, or by photocoagulation and laser through the dilated pupil. Most surgeons drain the subretinal fluid by perforating the sclera and the choroid so that the retina can settle back against the choroid. Synthetic materials such as silicone and teflon are used outside the sclera or within the scleral lamellae to achieve a scleral buckle. This shortens the globe and establishes contact between the choroid and the retina.

PROGNOSIS: Successful surgery reattaches the retina in 75% - 80% of the cases. An additional 10% can be cured with reoperation. The final visual acuity is unpredictable and unrelated to the anatomic reattachment of the retina. However, immediate surgery may restore excellent vision even when the macular area is detached. The patient may return to normal activity gradually, six weeks after successful surgery. Physical activity, especially quick head motions, should be restricted for a few weeks after surgery.

POISONING

A wide collection of organic substances, some of which are used in industry, may cause considerable visual damage, many of them causing rapid deterioration of vision. These substances include the alcohols, especially methyl alcohol, halogens, and certain aromatic amino and nitro-compounds. Their action is on the ganglion cells of the retina or on the optic nerve fibers, causing either contraction of the peripheral field or central visual field defects, or a combination of both.

There is evidence that in some cases a vascular disturbance is the initial cause. In others, the damage is neurogenic. Pathologically, the action of poisons is not well understood at present.

Ophthalmoscopic examination reveals edema of the retina and the optic disc. Occasionally, scattered hemorrhages may be seen in the retina. As the primary goal of this book is to describe ophthalmologic emergencies, we will discuss only those poisons which cause acute visual disturbances.

METHYL ALCOHOL (WOOD SPIRIT, CH_3OH)

Methyl alcohol taken orally is the most common route of poisoning. Drinking only a few milliliters of methyl alcohol may produce blindness. In industrial plants poisoning may occur also by inhalation of methyl alcohol fumes. Blindness caused by cutaneous absorption is rare, but such cases have been reported.

SIGNS AND SYMPTOMS: The general symptoms of methyl alcohol acute poisoning are nausea, vomiting, abdominal pain, headache, and dizziness. Delirium, convulsions, and stupor may occur in severe cases.

Blindness may be sudden, complete, and permanent shortly after poisoning. In certain cases, blindness is noticed on the second or third day after the ingestion of methyl alcohol. Ophthalmoscopic examination may reveal swelling of the optic disc, retinal edema, and dilatation of veins.

TREATMENT: Repeated gastric lavage during the first few days removes the methyl alcohol from the body. This is necessary because there is evidence that the methyl alcohol in the system continuously returns to the stomach.

Large amounts of ethyl alcohol given every few hours will protect the body against the toxic effects of methanol. This is due to preferential oxidation of ethyl alcohol by alcohol oxidase. The enzyme system is saturated with ethyl alcohol while the methyl alcohol is excreted. Ethyl alcohol treatment should be continued for a few days.

PROGNOSIS: In less severe cases, marked improvement may occur 4-6 weeks after poisoning. Reduced visual acuity and paracentral or cecocentral scotoma are the usual final results.

HALOGENATED HYDROCARBONS

Idoform (CHI_3) may cause loss of central vision with peripheral defect. Ophthalmoscopic changes are absent in most cases. The vision may return after discontinuance of the drug. The time of recovery varies from a few days to several months.

Methyl chloride (CH_3Cl) may cause retrobulbar neuritis, diplopia, and accommodation disturbances. Methyl bromide (CH_3Br) causes also acute visual loss. Both agents enter the human body by inhalation. Carbon tetrachloride ($C Cl_4$) and trichlorethylene ($CHCl:CCl_2$) rarely cause, if at all, sudden deterioration or loss of vision.

TREATMENT: The treatment is mainly preventive. No effective antidote is known for poisoning by halogenated hydrocarbons.

DRUGS

Chloramphenicol ($C_{11}H_{12}Cl_2N_2O_5$) is known to cause complete loss of vision after long-term administration in high doses. Most commonly, the loss of vision is due to optic neuritis or retrobulbar neuritis. Immediate discontinuation of the drug is imperative. The prognosis concerning vision is unpredictable.

Sulphanilamide ($C_6H_4(NH_2)SO_2NH_2$) occasionally may cause transient blindness. As only a few cases have been reported, not much is known about this kind of poisoning.

Quinine ($C_{20}H_{24}N_2O_2 + 3H_2O$) and Quinidine ($C_{20}H_{24}N_2O_2$). Quinine is still used as an antimalarial and antipyretic drug. Its use is widely spread also for criminal abortion. Quinidine is used mainly in cardiology. Toxic effects are reported mainly from the use of quinine. The pathogenesis of quinine poisoning is not completely understood.

General symptoms include confusion of speech, tinnitus, deafness, loss of consciousness, delirium, and coma. Ocular symptom is sudden loss or severe deterioration of vision.

Visual disturbances may occur after a single dose of the drug or after its prolonged administration. Visual disturbances are always bilateral, acute in nature, and of sudden onset. Vision may deteriorate rapidly and complete blindness is not unusual. The pupils are widely dilated.

Fundus examination reveals contracted arteries and edematous retina. Occasionally, the picture of complete occlusion of the central retinal artery can be seen, with a cherry red spot at the macula. Quinine poisoning may be confused with hysteria; in such cases, the appearance of the fundus is the deciding factor whether it is quinine poisoning or hysteria.

TREATMENT: The treatment is directed to produce vasodilatation. Retrobulbar injection of acetylcholine (200 mg), intravenous papaverine (50 mg every 3-4 hours), and amyl nitrate (repeated inhalations), and priscoline 25 mg t. i. d. , are among the most commonly used vasodilators. Treatment should be started immediately after making the diagnosis. Administration of vasodilators should be continued for several days at least.

PROGNOSIS: If the poisoning is not severe, vision may return in a few hours. In severe cases blindness may persist for several weeks. Permanent blindness has not been reported. Varying degrees of peripheral visual field contraction is the usual end result. Central vision is the least affected. Optic atrophy is common after quinine poisoning.

Filix Mas is an anthelmintic drug, rarely used in modern medicine. The toxic dose varies from individual to individual. The drug-induced symptoms (loss of vision) may appear on the first to the 12th day after administration of the drug. The condition may be unilateral. Loss of vision could be temporary or permanent. Ophthalmoscopy reveals constriction of retinal arteries and edema of the retina in most cases. Treatment consists of various vasodilators, as described for quinine poisoning.

The prognosis of filix mas poisoning is worse than that of quinine poisoning. The end result is often constricted visual fields and optic atrophy.

Ergot taken in massive doses as an abortifacient may cause temporary amblyopia. Ergot derivatives used in obstetrics occasionally also can cause temporary deterioration of vision. General symptoms include numbness in the limbs, often followed by gangrene or convulsions. Ophthalmologic symptoms are reduced vision and peripheral contraction of the visual fields. Fundus examination reveals severe vasoconstriction and edema of the retina. The treatment is directed to produce vasodilatation. The amblyopia is transient and optic atrophy does not occur.

Salicylates and Aspirin: Salicylates and aspirin in large doses may cause temporary amblyopia. It is not clear whether the loss of vision originates in the central nervous system or if it is due to a toxic effect on the ganglion cells.

General symptoms include tinnitus and deafness. Ophthalmologic symptoms, other than deteriorated vision, may include nystagmus, dilated pupils, and marked constriction of visual fields. Fundus examination often reveals constricted vessels of the retina.

Treatment should be concentrated on prevention of salicylate poisoning. Gastric lavage during the first few hours after salicylate or aspirin ingestion may reduce further absorption of the drug. Recovery is usually rapid. Permanent damage of vision is unusual.

GLAUCOMA

Sudden loss of vision due to glaucoma is discussed in the chapter on glaucoma.

CHORIORETINITIS AT THE MACULA

Acute chorioretinitis at the macula area may destroy useful vision within several days (Fig. 2-7). Therefore, the patient suffering from this type of inflammation may show up as an emergency case. The vast majority of inflammatory changes are endogenous in origin. Actually, there is not much difference between the etiology of chorioretinitis at the macula and of that elsewhere in the fundus. Toxoplasmosis, histoplasmosis, organismal metastasis from distant bacterial and viral infections and autoimmunologic reactions should be considered when visual deterioration occurs due to chorioretinitis (or retino-choroiditis) at the macula. However, it should be noted that in the overwhelming majority of cases of chorioretinitis the etiology cannot be determined.

SIGNS AND SYMPTOMS: In addition to the deterioration of vision, the patient may complain of pain or heaviness of the eye. On examination, the anterior segment of the eye may not show any sign of inflammation. Examination with an ophthalmoscope reveals cloudy vitreous and a yellowish-white patch at the posterior pole. The lesion is usually slightly elevated and, occasionally, a small hemorrhage may accompany the lesion.

DIFFERENTIAL DIAGNOSIS: If a cloudy vitreous is observed when examining a patient suffering from sudden deterioration of vision, the possibility of hemorrhage or inflammation, or both, should always be considered. Sometimes it is extremely difficult to differentiate between these two conditions.

TREATMENT: The treatment of chorioretinitis at the posterior pole is an absolute emergency. As laboratory test results are often disappointing, the ophthalmologist should immediately start non-specific therapy of chorioretinitis before laboratory results are known. This therapy is systemic corticosteroids (prednisone) in relatively large doses. The amount of medication depends on the severity of the lesion. Forty to 120 mg of prednisone per day is the starting dose if a vital structure such as the macula is involved.

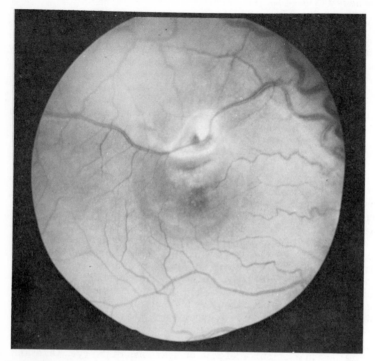

Fig. 2-7. Acute chorioretinitis at the macula. (Presumed histo-plasmic chorioretinitis.) The vision was 20/400.

Contraindications for steroids such as tuberculosis, peptic ulcer, diabetes should all be considered when one starts systemic steroid treatment, but hesitation and delayed treatment may compromise the final visual result.

Many ophthalmologists prefer to perform extensive laboratory investigation prior to any treatment. Skin tests for tuberculosis, histoplasmosis, complement fixation tests, methylene blue dye test (toxoplasmosis), x-ray pictures of chest and skull, CBC, and sedimentation rate are among the more common laboratory tests used to determine the etiology.

Topical treatment (also nonspecific) are cycloplegics (Cyclogyl 1%, Atropine 1%) and topical steroid drops (Inflamase forte, Prednefrin forte, Decadron). These drugs help also to reduce the active symptoms of the disease and also the retinal scarring. Also, topical treatment should start immediately.

The above-mentioned nonspecific emergency treatment may be changed or reconsidered once the results of the laboratory tests are available.

RETINAL HEMORRHAGE AT THE MACULA

Retinal hemorrhages may occur at the macular area and reduce visual acuity (Fig. 2-8). The decrease of vision may be abrupt or gradual. Hemorrhages may appear in association with systemic disease such as leukemia, anemia, thrombocytopenia, diabetes mellitus, hypertension, or ocular diseases such as high myopia, macular degeneration, or chorioretinitis. Among young adults, hemorrhage may occur in the absence of any detectable systemic or ocular disorder.

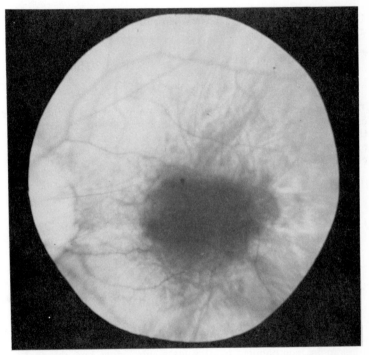

Fig. 2-8. Hemorrhage at the macula in a highly myopic eye

SIGNS AND SYMPTOMS: The patient's main complaint is abrupt or gradual deterioration of vision. The loss of vision is usually painless. No pathology is seen in the anterior segment. On fundus examination, different kinds of ophthalmoscopic pictures can be observed. If the hemorrhage appears as a macular star, the blood cells are in Henle's layer. If the hemorrhage is "boat-shaped," it is located between the nerve fibers and the internal limiting membrane of the retina (also called preretinal hemorrhage). Macular hemorrhage in high myopia may appear as a dark oval mass. In this case, the hemorrhage is deep and may be partly behind the pigment epithelium.

During absorption hemorrhages change their appearance. The color becomes rusty red, the size is smaller, and its shape is fragmented.

PROGNOSIS: Hemorrhage at the macula may take several weeks to clear; however, the prognosis of vision is relatively good in most cases, and return of full vision occurs quite often. On fundus examination there is no trace of the hemorrhage. In the case of high myopia, blood absorbs slowly and it may be replaced by organized exudate or a mass of pigment.

TRAUMA

Trauma can cause sudden loss or deterioration of vision in three ways:

1. Injury to the eyeball
2. Injury to the optic nerve
3. Injury to the central nervous system

The management of injury to the eyeball is described in the chapter on trauma, injury to the optic nerve is discussed in the chapter on trauma to the optic nerve, while injury to the central nervous system is discussed in the chapter on neuro-ophthalmologic emergencies.

BIBLIOGRAPHY

1. Av-Shalom, A., Berson, D., Gombos, G. M.: Michaelson, I. C. and Zauberman, H.: Some comments on the incidence of idiopathic retinal detachment among Africans. Amer J Ophthal 64: 384, 1967.

2. Ballantyne, A. J. and Michaelson, I. C.: The Fundus of the Eye. Williams and Wilkins, Baltimore, 1970.

3. Benson, W. E. and Spalter, H. F.: Vitreous hemorrhage. Surv Ophthal 15:297, 1971.

4. Cox, M. S., Schepens, C. L. and Freeman, H. M.: Retinal detachment due to ocular contusion. Arch Ophthal 76:678, 1966.

5. Dufour, D., Constantinioles, G. and Wannebroucq, C.: Action de la thrombosamine-heparine dans une thrombose arterielle retinienne. Bull Soc Ophtal Franc 68:137, 1968.

6. Duke-Elder, S.: System of Ophthalmology. Injuries. Vol. XIV. Mosby, St. Louis, 1972.

7. Duke-Elder, S. and Dobree, G. H. : System of Ophthalmology. Diseases of the Retina. Vol. 10. Mosby, St. Louis, 1967.

8. Dufour, R. : The pathogenesis of retinal detachment. Ophthalmologica 148:386, 1964.

9. Ellis, C. J. et al. : Medical investigation of retinal vascular occlusion. Brit Med J 2:1093, 1964.

10. Everett, W. G. : Bilateral retinal detachment and degenerations. Trans Amer Ophthal Soc 64:543, 1966.

11. Gall, J. : ACTH and cortisone administration in inducing the reabsorption of vitreous and retinal hemorrhages. Orv Hetil 101:1681, 1960.

12. Gombos, G. M. : A new treatment of central retinal artery occlusion. Ann Ophthal 2:893, 1970.

13. Hannon, J. F. : Vitreous hemorrhages associated with sickle-cell hemoglobin C disease. Amer J Ophthal 42:707, 1956.

14. Hardenbergh, F. E. : Occlusion of central retinal artery. Arch Ophthal 67:556, 1962.

15. Hawkey, C. and Howell, M. : Intravenous streptokinase in the treatment of retinal vascular occlusion. J Clin Path 17:363, 1964.

16. Klien, B. A. : Prevention of retinal venous occlusion with special reference to ambulatory dicumarol therapy. Amer J Ophthal 33:175, 1950.

17. Lanske, R. K. : Central retinal artery occlusion. Amer J Ophthal 60:716, 1965.

18. Lincoff, H. , McLean, J. M. and Nano, H. : Cryosurgical treatment of retinal detachment. Trans Amer Acad Ophthal Otolaryng 68:412, 1964.

19. Meyer-Schwickerath, G. : Indications and limitations of light coagulations of the retina. Trans Amer Acad Ophthal Otolaryng 63:725, 1959.

20. Paton, B. , Rubinstein, K. and Smith, V. R. : Arterial insufficiency in the occlusion of retina venous occlusion. Trans Ophthal Soc U. K. 84:559, 1964.

21. Radnót, M. and Follmann, P. : Rheomacrodex dextran in the treatment of the occlusion of the central retinal vein. Ann Ophthal 1:58, 1969.

22. Rubinstein, K. : Arterial insufficiency in retinal venous occlusion. Trans Ophthal Soc U. K. 85:564, 1964.

23. Schepens, C. L. , Okamura, I. D. and Brockhurst, R. J. : The scleral buckling procedures. Arch Ophthal 58:797, 1957.

24. Welch, R. B. and Goldberg, M. F. : Sickle-cell hemoglobin and its relation to fundus abnormality. Arch Ophthal 75:353, 1966.

25. Wise, G. N. , Dollery, C. T. and Henkind, P. : The Retinal Circulation. Harper and Row, New York, 1971.

CHAPTER 3

EMERGENCIES DUE TO INFECTIONS OR INFLAMMATIONS

Ophthalmic emergencies due to infection or inflammation, which the physician may encounter in the emergency room or in his office, can be divided into three groups, infection or inflammation of:

      I. the eyelids and the lacrimal system
     II. the orbit
    III. the eyeball, including the conjunctiva

The signs, symptoms, and treatment of the infection or inflammation is somewhat different for each group.

I. INFECTIONS OF THE EYELIDS AND LACRIMAL SYSTEM

DACRYOCYSTITIS

Dacryocystitis is an infection of the lacrimal sac. The disease may appear in the acute or in the chronic form. Only acute dacryocystitis is a real emergency and, though it generally occurs unilaterally, it may appear bilaterally. Dacryocystitis occurs when there is an obstruction of the nasolacrimal duct. The etiologic causes are bacterial or mycotic. Staphylococcus pyogenes, Diplococcus pneumoniae or Hemophilus influenzae are the more common bacteria which cause dacryocystitis. Candida albicans causes chronic dacryocystitis; however, occasionally, the chronic form of dacryocystitis may flare up and appear in its acute form. Delayed canalization of the nasolacrimal ducts is a very common cause of dacryocystitis in infants.

SIGNS AND SYMPTOMS: Acute dacryocystitis, which may appear in the emergency room, is painful. The lacrimal sac area is swollen, the skin over the sac is red and tender. Purulent material can be expressed from the sac. The latter is important in the diagnosis, since sinus tumor or mucoceles may cause a similar appearance. Chronic dacryocystitis causes tearing. Mucopurulent material can usually be expressed from the lacrimal sac.

LABORATORY EXAMINATIONS: Purulent material expressed from the lacrimal sac should be examined. The etiologic agent can be identified microscopically from a stained smear. A culture and sensitivity test is helpful to choose the most suitable antibiotic to be used.

TREATMENT: Acute dacryocystitis should be treated with systemic antibiotics. Penicillin, 1-2 million units daily, intramuscularly, or ampicillin, 2 grams daily, orally or intramuscularly (500 mg every 6 hours), or tetracycline, 1 gram daily (250 mg every 6 hours), should be administered for one week. Warm compresses applied to the inflamed area 4-5 times a day is a helpful adjunct in the treatment of an acute dacryocystitis. Direct irrigation of the lacrimal sac with antibiotic solution is advocated by a few ophthalmologists.

Chronic dacryocystitis does not require immediate attention. The nasolacrimal duct obstruction which causes the infection should be relieved by probing. If this is unsuccessful, surgery should be performed at a later date. In the infant, probing of the nasolacrimal duct is indicated when the duct fails to open and the sac becomes infected.

PROGNOSIS: Acute dacryocystitis responds favorably to antibiotic treatment. Recurrences are common. Perforation of the skin and fistula formation also may occur.

FINAL TREATMENT: Definite treatment is required after the acute infection subsides. Free drainage into the nose should be restored either by probing through the nasolacrimal duct or by surgery, creating a new opening between the lacrimal sac and the nose. This procedure is called dacryocystorhinostomy.

DACRYOADENITIS

Dacryoadenitis is an acute inflammation of the lacrimal gland. The etiologic agent could be viral or bacterial. Dacryoadenitis may be seen in children as a complication of measles, mumps, or influenza. Dacryoadenitis may develop in association with gonorrhea infection, sarcoidosis, tuberculosis, lymphatic leukemia, or lymphosarcoma. In the latter four conditions, the inflammation is chronic rather than acute.

SIGNS AND SYMPTOMS: Acute dacryoadenitis causes pain at the upper temporal aspect of the orbit and the corresponding area is swollen.

TREATMENT: Warm compresses and analgesics are required as unspecific treatments. If bacterial infection is suspected, a tetracycline, 1 gram daily, or another broad-spectrum antibiotic in equivalent amounts should be used. Incision of the gland is indicated only if definite pus collection is present. Dacryoadenitis due to sarcoidosis or leukemia should be treated with a steroid such as prednisone, 30-40 mg daily.

HORDEOLUM (STY)

Hordeolum is a localized staphylococcal infection of the glands of the eyelid. There are two types:

1. External hordeolum
2. Internal hordeolum

External hordeolum involves the glands of Zeis and Moll. The center of the infection is the lash follicle. This type of hordeolum is not too painful. The pain is localized at the site of the infection. The edema of the eyelid is moderate. The infection very often drains externally.

Internal hordeolum is the other type of acute infection which involves the meibomian gland of the tarsus. This type of hordeolum is much more painful and the edema of the eyelid is more pronounced. General signs of inflammation such as leucocytosis or fever are not very common.

TREATMENT: Treatment of hordeolum includes:

1. Local antibiotics
2. Warm compresses

Any antibiotic ointment can be used in the conjunctival sac. Chloromycetin, 1% or tetracycline, 1% or erythromycin, 1% eye ointments, will cure the infection equally as well and will prevent spreading of the infection. Warm compresses of either boiled water or a 3% boric acid solution should be applied for 10-15 minutes, 3-4 times a day.

Incising or squeezing a hordeolum is unnecessary and is not recommended because it quite likely will spread the infection.

CHALAZION, INFECTED CHALAZION

Chalazion is a chronic granulomatous inflammation of the meibomian or Zeis gland (Fig. 3-1). It may follow a hordeolum. It is a localized swelling of the eyelid. In general, this is not a painful condition and rarely is seen in the emergency room. Occasionally it can be inflamed, appearing as an "inflamed chalazion." The immediate treatment is the same as described for hordeolum. Surgical excision of the chalazion is indicated at a later stage, after the acute inflammation has subsided.

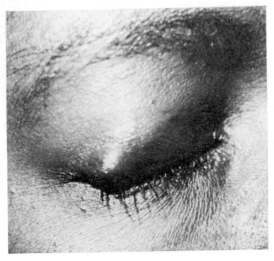

Fig. 3-1. Infected chalazion

II. INFECTION OF THE ORBIT

ORBITAL CELLULITIS

Orbital cellulitis rarely occurs as a primary disease. Generally, it results from an infection in the sinuses, especially in the ethmoid bone. Rarely, the infection is blood-borne. Pneumococci, streptococci, staphylococci are the most common bacteria but gram negative bacteria, virus, or fungus are also among the organisms that cause orbital infection.

SIGNS AND SYMPTOMS: Swelling, redness of the eyelid, chemosis of the conjunctiva, proptosis of the globe, and pain around and behind the eyeball are the usual signs of orbital cellulitis (Fig. 3-2). Muscular movements may be painful and limited or completely absent according to the severeness of the disease. The visual acuity is reduced. Fundus examination occasionally may reveal blurred disc or intraocular hemorrhage, due most likely to the pressure behind the eye. Leucocytosis, fever, and malaise generally accompany the local symptoms.

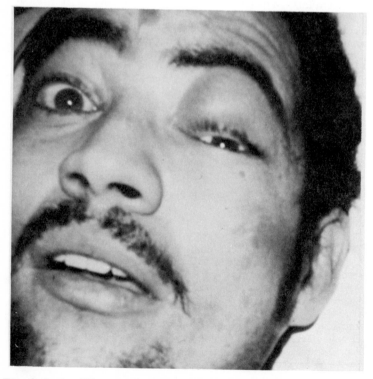

Fig. 3-2. A mild case of orbital cellulitis. Laboratory results revealed growth of hemophilus influenzae.

In severe cases of orbital infection or inflammation the so-called superior orbital fissure syndrome or the orbital apex syndrome may be present. In cases of superior orbital fissure syndrome the inflammatory process involves the III, IV, V-1, and VI cranial nerves entering the orbit at the superior orbital fissure, inhibiting and, in more severe cases, severing their functions. The pathologic process of the orbital apex syndrome involves the optic nerve as well as the III, IV, V-1, VI cranial nerves. Many times one cannot differentiate between these two syndromes.

DIFFERENTIAL DIAGNOSIS: Orbital cellulitis must be differentiated from unilateral exophthalmos due to other causes. Orbital tumors with secondary infection must be ruled out.

TREATMENT: Antibiotics in large doses must be administered intravenously or intramuscularly. Penicillin 20 million units per day I. V. and a broad-spectrum antibiotic such as Cephalothin 4. 0 gm/day I. V. or gentamicin (Garamycin) 100 mg/day I. M. are not unusual dosages. One should recall that insufficient treatment may not stop the spreading of the disease which may extend, causing cavernous sinus thrombosis, meningitis, brain abscess, orbital periostitis, panophthalmitis, or optic neuritis. In addition to the antibiotic treatment, warm compresses are helpful to localize the inflammatory reaction.

Surgery of the involved sinus or the orbit is not recommended as it may spread the infection and cause unnecessary complications. Surgical drainage or exploration is indicated only if the condition worsens steadily for a few days. Surgery is definitely not required in the emergency room.

CAVERNOUS SINUS THROMBOSIS

Cavernous sinus thrombosis occurs mainly as a result of blood-borne infection from the throat, nasal cavities, or the facial area. Spreading of an orbital cellulitis is also a common cause of cavernous sinus thrombosis. Most often, streptococcus bacteria is the etiologic agent.

SIGNS AND SYMPTOMS: The general signs of disease are fever (sometimes septic type), chills, somnolence, headache, and, occasionally, nausea and vomiting. Marked leucocytosis is present.

DIFFERENTIAL DIAGNOSIS: Sometimes it is difficult to differentiate between orbital cellulitis with orbital apex involvement and cavernous sinus thrombosis. In orbital involvement, the pupillary reflexes remain normal. Blurred disc or papilledema are more common in cavernous sinus thrombosis than in orbital cellulitis. The involvement of the II, III, IV, V-1, and VI cranial nerves are more pronounced in cavernous sinus thrombosis than in orbital apex syndrome. The most important difference between the two diseases is that in the case of cavernous sinus thrombosis the patient is in a far more toxic general condition.

TREATMENT: The administration of antibiotics in massive dosages is a life-saving procedure. Penicillin and Cephalothin must be administered intravenously. Twenty million units of penicillin and 4.0 gm of Cephalothin per day are not exaggerated doses. Gentamicin (Garamycin) 120 mg/day (30 mg every 6 hours) should be administered I.M. The administration of a synthetic penicillin such as ampicillin in amounts of 4-8 grams per day should also be considered. If the patient is not nauseous, and one of the above-mentioned antibiotics cannot be administered for any reason, chloramphenicol, 2 gm/day (500 mg 4 times a day) by mouth can be added to the treatment. This medication must be continued until positive culture sensitivity tests indicate the use of other antibiotics.

III. INFECTIONS AND INFLAMMATIONS OF THE EYEBALL AND THE CONJUNCTIVA

A. CONJUNCTIVITIS

One of the more common eye diseases is conjunctivitis -- inflammation of the conjunctiva. The conjunctiva is an exposed tissue and, regardless of its defense mechanism, inflammation may occur very often. Special defense mechanisms include: a) the mechanical washing by tears of the conjunctival debris and microorganism into the nose, and b) the lysozyme content of the tear solution which reduces the growth of bacteria and other organisms in the conjunctival sac. Most cases of conjunctivitis are not absolute "emergency" but only "urgent." However, occasionally conjunctivitis may cause serious complications by the microorganism invading the cornea (gonococcal conjunctivitis). Conjunctivitis can be classified according to etiologic factors as follows:

1. Bacterial
2. Viral
3. Fungal
4. Parasitic
5. Allergic
6. Unknown etiology

1. Bacterial infection can be caused by cocci or bacilli, both gram positive and gram negative organisms. The bacteria involved more commonly include the following:

a) Staphylococcus pyogenes (aureus)
b) Streptococcus viridans
c) Diplococcus pneumoniae
d) Corynebacterium diphtheriae
e) Neissieria gonorrhoeae
f) Hemophilus influenzae
g) Hemophilus conjunctivitidis (Koch-Weeks bacillus)
h) Moraxella lacunata
i) Pasteurella tularensis
j) Pseudomonas aeruginosa
k) Microbacillus polymorphicus necroticans
l) Proteus vulgaris

2. Viruses causing conjunctivitis are the following:

   a) Epidemic keratoconjunctivitis (EKC). (Adenovirus type 8)
   b) Adenoviruses 3 and 7
   c) Herpes simplex
   d) Molluscum contagiosum
   e) Newcastle virus
   f) Lymphogranuloma venereum
   g) Trachoma
   h) Inclusion blennorrhea
   i) Measles
   j) German measles
   k) Cat scratch fever
   l) Mumps
   m) Variola
   n) Varicella
   o) Vaccinia

3. Fungal infection of the conjunctiva is not a common cause of conjunctivitis. The more common fungi include the following:

   a) Actinomyces
   b) Aspergillus
   c) Blastomyces
   d) Candida
   e) Coccidioides
   f) Nocardia
   g) Phycomycetes (mucormycosis)
   h) Rhinosporidium
   i) Sporotrichum

4. Parasitic infection of the conjunctiva could be caused by:

   a) Onchocerca caecutiens (volvulus)
   b) Loa loa
   c) Wuchereria bancrofti
   d) Nematoda
   e) Trematoda
   f) Cestoda
   g) Thelazia (Californiensis-Callipaeda)
   h) Trypanosoma
   i) Arthropoda

5. Allergic types of conjunctivitis are the following:

   a) Atopic conjunctivitis
   b) Microbiallergic conjunctivitis
   c) Allergic dermatoconjunctivitis
   d) Vernal conjunctivitis

6. Conjunctivitis of unknown etiology are the following:

   a) Follicular conjunctivitis

  b) Ocular rosacea
  c) Ocular pemphigus
  d) Erythema multiforme
  e) Epidermolysis bullosa
  f) Psoriasis
  g) Reiter's disease
  h) Keratoconjunctivitis sicca

SIGNS AND SYMPTOMS: Conjunctivitis is not a painful eye disease. Discharge, tearing, and itching may occur. Although the eye is red, the vision is not impaired. Most types of conjunctivitis are bilateral. The disease usually starts in one eye and spreads to the other eye.

The following table may be helpful in the diagnosis of the different types of conjunctivitis.

	Discharge	Tearing	Injection	Itching
VIRAL	±	+ + +	+ +	+
BACTERIAL	+ + +	+	+ +	+
FUNGAL	±	±	+	-
PARASITIC	±	±	+	-
ALLERGIC	±	+	+ +	+ + +

LABORATORY EXAMINATIONS: Stained smear taken from the conjunctival fornix is useful in differentiating the causal agent of conjunctivitis. In viral conjunctivitis, monocytes will be found on the smear. In bacterial conjunctivitis, bacteria and polymorphonuclear cells are expected. In fungal infection, occasional hyphae can be found (stained with KOH). When allergic conjunctivitis is present, eosinophils are the most common findings.

TREATMENT: Viral conjunctivitis is treated with topical decongestant drops containing naphazoline, such as Albalon or Vasocon, and instillation of sulfonamide or an antibiotic ointment such as Neomycin, Polymycin, Bacitracin, Chloromycetin, Aureomycin, or Terramycin. Decongestant eye drops relieve the acute symptoms of redness and heaviness. Sulfa or antibiotics are helpful in cases where the infection is caused by a large virus. Sulfa, Aureomycin, and Terramycin also are very useful in the treatment of trachoma. Although antibiotics are not effective in the treatment of small viruses, their use is recommended to prevent secondary bacterial invasion.

Bacterial conjunctivitis is treated with broad-spectrum antibiotic drops or ointment. Good medical management of bacterial conjunctivitis includes examination of a stained smear and a culture taken before starting any medication. Chloromycetin, Aureomycin, Terramycin, Neomycin, Bacitracin, and Garamycin are antibiotics effective against most types of bacterial infection. If after 3-4 days the treatment is ineffective, the medication should be changed according to the sensitivity of the culture taken initially.

Fungal conjunctivitis is treated with amphotericin B (Fungizone), 0. 15% solution. Drops should be instilled into the conjunctival sac every hour. If the causal agent is Candida albicans, the conjunctivitis may respond to nystatin (Mycostatin) ointment, 100,000 units/gm. Instillation of ointment is necessary at least 4 times a day.

The treatment of conjunctivitis due to parasites depends upon the causative agent. Onchocerca volvulus, or loa loa must be treated by systemic chemotherapy with diethylcarbamazine (Hetrazan). Other parasites such as larvae of Ascaris or ocular myiasis must be removed mechanically.

Allergic conjunctivitis is treated with topical corticosteroids such as prednisone, prednisolone, or dexamethasone eyedrops (Inflamase, Decadron, Vasocidin, Prednefrin forte). Cool clean air is beneficial. Cold water compresses may relieve acute symptoms. Prolonged steroid treatment may precipitate secondary bacterial infection; therefore, topical antibiotics should be considered.

Topical steroids also can cause elevated intraocular pressure when it is applied for long periods of time.

Most conjunctivitis of unknown origin has no specific treatment. Artificial tears (Tearosol) are helpful if the tear production is insufficient, as in keratoconjunctivitis sicca. Local or systemic steroids may be helpful in erythema multiforme bullosum. Mild decongestant eyedrops containing naphazoline, 0. 05% or 0. 1% (Vasocon or Albalon) may relieve acute symptoms.

CONJUNCTIVITIS IN THE NEWBORN
(OPHTHALMIA NEONATORUM)

Conjunctivitis in the newborn is an acute emergency. At one time, the term neonatorum was reserved for ocular gonorrheal infections in the newborn. However, now it is used to describe any acute purulent conjunctivitis occurring in the first two weeks of life. The cause of the conjunctivitis could be:

1. Iatrogenic (chemical after instillation of silver nitrite solution)
2. Bacterial (gonococcus, staphylococcus, pneumococcus)
3. Viral (inclusion conjunctivitis)

Because of the prophylaxis required by law, neonatal conjunctivitis due to gonorrhea is rare in the United States. Today it occurs in less than 0. 03% of the newborn. Other bacterial conjunctivitis may occur also in early infancy. Bacteria which are most common are staphylococcus, streptococcus, hemophilus influenzae, pneumococcus, and coliform organisms.

Viral conjunctivitis, also called inclusion conjunctivitis or inclusion blennorrhea, is caused by a large atypical virus which belongs to the psittacosis-lymphogranuloma venereum-trachoma group. This virus often inhabits the genitourinary system and passes to the infant's conjunctiva during delivery.

SIGNS AND SYMPTOMS: The signs of conjunctivitis in the newborn are more pronounced than those of adult conjunctivitis. The conjunctivitis is usually bilateral. The lids are swollen; exudation and pus formation are seen all around the palpebral fissures. The conjunctiva is chemotic and beefy. In neglected cases, corneal involvement may occur and presents as corneal opacity, ulceration, or even perforation of the cornea.

DIAGNOSIS: The time of onset is an important factor in diagnosis. The following table may be helpful to establish the diagnosis.

TIME OF ONSET	CAUSING FACTOR
1 - 2 days	Silver nitrate
1 - 5 days	Gonococcus (Staphylococcus pneumococcus?)
5 - 10 days	Inclusion conjunctivitis
11 - 21 days	Staphylococcus, pneumococcus, or other bacteria

A laboratory examination is the best way to differentiate the causative factor of conjunctivitis. In bacterial conjunctivitis, microscopic examination of stained material from the conjunctiva will reveal gram negative cocci (gonorrhea) or gram positive cocci (diplococcus pneumoniae of staphylococcus). In inclusion conjunctivitis, basophilic cytoplasmic inclusion bodies in the epithelial cells can be found in Giemsa stained smears. The predominant inflammatory cells in the exudate are polymorphonuclear leucocytes.

When conjunctivitis is caused by silver nitrate, neither bacteria nor inclusion bodies are expected on stained conjunctival scrapings. Routine cultures should be taken under either condition regardless if the specific cause is in doubt or is clinically evident.

PREVENTIVE MEASURES: Gonococcal conjunctivitis may be prevented by instilling silver nitrate solution, 1%, into the conjunctival sac. In some states this prophylaxis is still legally required. Another preventive measure is the instillation of penicillin ointment, 100,000 units/gm, into the conjunctival sac.

TREATMENT: The treatment of gonococcal conjunctivitis is the frequent instillation of penicillin ointment, 100,000 units/gm for several days, until all signs of infection disappear. Many ophthalmologists use erythromycin (Erythrocin, Ilotycine) or tetracycline (Aureomycin, Terramycin, Achromycin) rather than penicillin.

If the ophthalmia neonatorum is due to virus (inclusion conjunctivitis), the choice of treatment is broad-spectrum antibiotics such as tetracycline (Aureomycin, Terramycin, Achromycin) or sulfonamides (Gantrisin), or both. Topical administration of these medications, at least four times a day for one week to ten days, is a very effective treatment. If the silver nitrate conjunctivitis is severe, steroid drops with antibiotics is the correct treatment. The steroids reduce the inflammation and the antibiotics prevent secondary infection.

B. INFECTION OF THE CORNEA
KERATITIS AND CORNEAL ULCERS

Corneal infection is an extremely serious condition. Improper diagnosis and faulty management may result in significant visual impairment. Corneal infection can be caused by bacteria, virus, or fungus. Other possible causes of corneal inflammation or infection are vitamin "A" deficiency, hypersensitivity reaction, seventh nerve palsy-Bell's palsy (lagophthalmos), fifth nerve lesion (neurotrophic ulcer) and corneal ulcers (Mooren's ulcer) of unknown cause. Corneal infection can be superficial, affecting only the epithelium, or deep, involving the stroma. Corneal tissue is a very good culture medium for microorganism.

Corneal infection or ulcer can be caused by the following bacteria:

* Diplococcus pneumoniae
  Streptococcus hemolyticus
* Staphylococcus aureus
* Pseudomonas aeruginosa
  Moraxella lacunata
* Moraxella liquefaciens
  Klebsiella pneumoniae
  Hemophilus influenzae
  Escherichia coli
  Proteus vulgaris
  Brucella abortus
  Neisseria gonorrhoeae
  Neisseria meningitidis

* The four common pathogens.

Bacterial infection of the conjunctiva and the cornea may occur simultaneously. Most of the bacteria attack the cornea only if the epithelial layer is not intact. However, there are a few organisms which may attack the cornea even though the corneal epithelium is intact. These are:

Neisseria gonorrhoeae
Corynebacterium diphtheriae
Koch-Weeks bacilli

Viruses causing corneal lesions are as follows:

Herpes simplex
Herpes zoster

> Variola
> Vaccinia
> Epidemic keratoconjunctivitis

Fungi causing corneal lesions include the following:

> Candida albicans
> Actinomyces
> Aspergillus
> Blastomyces
> Phycomycetes (mucormycosis)
> Nocardia
> Sporotrichum

SIGNS AND SYMPTOMS: Pain and photophobia are the more common complaints of the patient who suffers from infection or inflammation of the cornea. The vision is reduced. The conjunctival vessels, as well as the deeper vessels, are dilated. This vessel dilatation causes a redness of the affected eye. As some degree of iritis always accompanies severe corneal involvement, the pupil is constricted.

If bacterial corneal ulcers are present, a light gray infiltration ring can be observed around a deepened area (the corneal ulcer).

Corneal lesion caused by herpes simplex virus appears as dendritic ulcer (Fig. 3-3). The dendritic ulcer stains green with fluorescein.

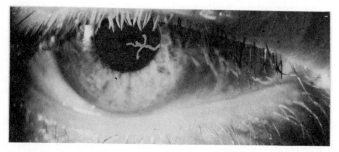

Fig. 3-3. Dendritic ulcer of the cornea

Fungal ulcers of the cornea are gray, indolent, and slowly progressive. They most often follow injury. They may develop as a complication of treatment of a wound with antibiotics or steroids for prolonged periods of time.

DIAGNOSIS: Corneal infection or inflammation must be differentiated from acute glaucoma (in which the pupil is dilated). The difference between conjunctivitis and corneal involvement depends upon the presence or absence of pain. Conjunctivitis is not painful, only discomfort is present. Corneal ulcer or inflammation is always accompanied with pain.

Laboratory examination is helpful in diagnosing bacterial infection. In most cases, the organism can be identified by a stained smear of the corneal scrapings. Cultures are necessary especially to achieve antibiotic sensitivity studies against the causative bacteria. If the infection is viral, the laboratory is not much help as neither the virus nor special cells can be seen on a stained smear. Herpes simplex virus can be identified by transferring corneal scrapings to the chorioallantoic membrane of the chick embryo and cultivating.

Hyphae of fungus can be found in corneal scrapings if fungal corneal ulcer is present. Special staining with KOH is necessary for this purpose.

Corneal ulcer (Mooren's ulcer) of unknown cause is a nonexudative ulcer near the limbus. The central edge of the border is elevated. Corneal scrapings do not show any microbes. Similar sterile ulcer, of unknown cause, may be present also in polyarteritis nodosa.

TREATMENT: Bacterial Infection. When bacteria is the cause, corneal infection requires early diagnosis and vigorous immediate treatment. Topical and subconjunctival application of antibiotics is indicated in most cases. Systemic antibiotics should be considered if the condition is advanced. If corneal infection is not too severe, frequent instillation of gentamicin solution 3 mg/cc (Garamycin) or ointment is necessary. This drug is effective against Gram positive cocci and Gram negative bacilli including pseudomonas. A combination of neomycin, polymyxin, and bacitracin (Neosporin) is also an effective treatment. Topical antibiotics should be used every hour. The irrigation of the conjunctival sac with sterile physiologic solution to remove pus and debris before instillation of antibiotics is a very useful adjunct. An eye with bacterial infection should not be bandaged since covering the eye promotes bacterial growth.

The broad-spectrum antibiotic treatment should be continued until laboratory results of culture and sensitivity are available. Change of antibiotic may be required according to the sensitivity test. A cyclopegic, such as Atropine 1% or Cyclogyl 1%, should also be employed 2-3 times a day since mild iritis is always present in cases of corneal infection, and synechiae are formed during the inflammatory process.

If the corneal infection is severe, subconjunctival administration of antibiotics is indicated. Not all kinds of antibiotics are recommended for subconjunctival use. Some antibiotics cause severe irritation and conjunctival necrosis. A synthetic penicillin, such as ampicillin or methicillin, is well tolerated by the conjunctiva and is effective against many infections. Ampicillin 100-250 mg, methicillin 200-500 mg, gentamicin (Garamycin) 20-40 mg, cephaloridine (Loridine) 50 mg, or cephalothin (Keflin) 50 mg is an adequate dose for subconjunctival use. Other antibiotics such as chloramphenicol or polymyxin, neomycin or tetracycline also can be used subconjunctivally; however, because of their tendency to cause severe irritation and necrosis of the conjunctiva, they should be reserved for special indications. Before subconjunctival injection, a topical anesthetic such as Dorsacain (benoxinate hydrochloride 0. 4%) or Ophthaine (proparacaine hydrochloride 0. 5%) drops should be instilled two or three times. Lidocaine (Xylocain), 2%, in amounts of 0. 2-0. 3cc should be injected together with the antibiotic to reduce further the patient's discomfort. Subconjunctival injections may be repeated twice a day if necessary. In severe cases of corneal infection, systemic administration of antibiotics is indicated. The use of systemic chloramphenicol in combination with one of the newer synthetic penicillins is advocated by many ophthalmologists. The acceptable dosage of these drugs for ophthalmologic use is as follows:

Chloramphenicol, 2. 0-3. 0 gram per day, and ampicillin, 1. 0-4. 0 grams per day, may be given either orally or intravenously. Against resistant staphylococci, methicillin up to 8 grams per day I. V. , or lincomycin (Lincocin), 2. 0-4. 0 grams per day I. V. , may provide adequate coverage. Gentamicin (Garamycin), 100 mg I. M. per day, or cephalexin (Keflex), 1-2 gm P. O. per day also are recommended medications.

Viral Infection of the Cornea: The most common viral infection of the cornea, herpes simplex, is treated with idoxuridine (IDU). Antiviral agents interfere with the normal viral synthesis of deoxyribonucleic acid. IDU (Herplex) is a 0. 1% solution and is administered to the affected eye every hour during the day, and every two hours at night. IDU is available also as an ointment (Stoxil). The ointment should be applied 4 to 5 times a day in a 24-hour period. Mechanical debridement of the corneal epithelium is also a very effective treatment in herpetic keratitis.

In addition to IDU or mechanical debridement of the corneal epithelium, a cycloplegic (Cyclogyl 1% or Homatropin 5%) and a topical antibiotic (Chloromycetin, Aureomycin, Terramycin, Neomycin or Garamycin) should be instilled three times a day to reduce secondary iritis and to prevent secondary bacterial infection.

Varicella and measle infections of the cornea are also treated with IDU, a cycloplegic, and a broad-spectrum topical antibiotic, as described for herpes simplex.

Herpes zoster infection is treated with a cycloplegic (Cyclogyl 1% or Homatropin 5%) 2 or 3 times a day. In severe cases, a systemic corticosteroid such as prednisone, 40 mg per day, is indicated. One must be certain of the diagnosis of herpes zoster before prescribing steroids since steroids may aggregate other viral diseases of the cornea.

Other viral diseases of the cornea should be treated with a cycloplegic and a broad-spectrum antibiotic as a first-aid measurement.

Mycotic infections of the cornea should be treated with amphotericin B (Fungizone), an antifungal agent. Amphotericin B eyedrops containing 4-10 mg per ml should be instilled into the conjunctival sac every hour or every two hours the first day. The instillation of amphotericin B 4-6 times a day is necessary for at least two weeks.

Subconjunctival administration is indicated in severe cases. The maximal dose is 60 micrograms in 0.5 ml solution which can be repeated daily. Systemic administration of amphotericin B is indicated only in selected cases because of the high toxicity of the drug.

Nystatin (Mycostatin) is an antibiotic which is effective against a few fungi, in particular against Candida albicans. Mycostatin is available in ointment form 100,000 units per mg. If the corneal infection is due to Candida albicans, Mycostatin ointment should be instilled into the conjunctival sac 4-6 times a day. Systemic administration of Mycostatin is not effective in corneal infection. In addition to the antifungal agent, a cycloplegic and a broad-spectrum antibiotic should also be used to reduce iridocyclitis and to prevent secondary bacterial infection. Recently, flucytosine, a potent antifungal medication was introduced against Candida albicans. The medication is given orally. The dosage is 200 mg/kg daily.

Phlyctenular keratitis responds dramatically to topical steroids and cycloplegics. Exposure keratitis or neuroparalytic keratitis is treated with a mild cycloplegic (Mydriacyl, 0.5%), an antibiotic and a lubricating agent (Tearosol) as a primary first-aid measurement.

The general rules concerning treatment of corneal infection are:

1. Prior to treatment, perform laboratory examinations.
2. Antibiotics are indicated in bacterial infection and are helpful in other infections to prevent secondary bacterial infection.
3. Cycloplegics are helpful to reduce iritis and, in this way, they relieve pain.
4. If the infection is bacterial or viral in origin, do not use topical steroids.
5. If bacterial infection is suspected, do not patch the eye.

C. UVEITIS

Inflammation of the uvea is called uveitis. One or all three portions of the uvea (iris, ciliary body, choroid) may be involved simultaneously. Iritis and iridocyclitis are often called anterior uveitis. Posterior uveitis is the inflammation of the choroid. Pan-uveitis is inflammation of all three parts of the uvea. Uveitis, anterior or posterior, may be unilateral or bilateral. Uveitis can be divided into two large groups:

A. Suppurative
B. Nonsuppurative
   a) Nongranulomatous uveitis
   b) Granulomatous uveitis

Other classifications are:

    a) Exogenous uveitis
    b) Endogenous uveitis

The causative agent can be either a foreign substance (or organism) or the result of a systemic process.

Woods outlined the etiology of granulomatous uveitis as follows:

A. Nonpyogenic microorganisms pathogenic for man:
    1. Syphilis
    2. Tuberculosis
    3. Brucellosis
    4. Leptospriosis
    5. Infections with other nonpyogenic organisms (leprosy)

B. Filterable viruses and rickettsia:
    1. Behcet's syndrome (uveitis with aphthous ulcers)
    2. Vogt-Koyanagi-Harada syndrome
    3. Herpes simplex virus
    4. Herpes zoster virus
    5. Lymphogranuloma venereum
    6. Undetermined and unknown viruses

C. Protozoan infections:
    1. Trypanosomiasis
    2. Toxoplasmosis

D. Fungus infections:
    1. Actinomycosis
    2. Blastomycosis
    3. Histoplasmosis
    4. Infection with other rare fungi

E. Helminth infection:
    1. Nematodes
    2. Onchocerciasis
    3. Ancylostoma larvae
    4. Cestodes
    5. Taenia echinococcus
    6. Cysticercus cellulosae
    7. Diptera larvae

F. Unknown agents:
    1. Sympathetic ophthalmia
    2. Sarcoidosis

Granulomatous uveitis follows a chronic low-grade clinical course. Remissions and exacerbations are common. Nongranulomatous uveitis is a more acute disease. The onset is acute and more intense, while the course is shorter.

A nongranulomatous uveitis may be associated with a febrile illness such as measles, mumps, or whooping cough. In these cases the uveitis is less severe and very often self-limited.

SIGNS AND SYMPTOMS: <u>Anterior uveitis.</u> The patient complains of (a) pain in the eye, (b) headache, (c) photophobia, and (d) blurred vision. The eye is injected, the conjunctival and the deep episcleral vessels around the limbus are dilated. The pupil is constricted and often irregular because of posterior synechiae. Examination with a slit lamp shows keratic precipitates on the inner surface of the cornea (Fig. 3-4). The keratic precipitates tend to be finer and discreet in nongranulomatous uveitis, and of a large mutton-fat type in granulomatous uveitis. Flare and cells are seen in the anterior chamber in both the granulomatous and nongranulomatous types. The intraocular pressure may be normal, low, or elevated. This depends upon (a) the aqueous formation (which is less in an inflamed eye), (b) posterior synechiae (impeding the flow of aqueous from the posterior chamber to the anterior chamber), and (c) function of chamber angle concerning aqueous outflow (which may be impaired in an inflamed eye).

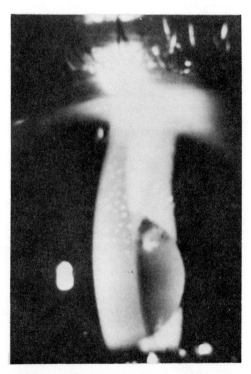

Fig. 3-4. Slit-lamp photography of the cornea shows keratic precipitates on the inner surface of the cornea.

Posterior uveitis: The pain and photophobia is less in posterior uveitis than in anterior uveitis. The vision is blurred because of vitreous haze. If the active lesion is in the posterior pole, the vision can be markedly reduced. On fundus examination, the lesion appears yellowish-white in color. The lesion can vary in size.

Anterior and posterior uveitis may appear simultaneously; therefore, careful examination of the anterior and posterior segments is always required.

DIFFERENTIAL DIAGNOSIS: Anterior uveitis must be differentiated from conjunctivitis and acute glaucoma. In conjunctivitis, the vision is normal, there is no pain or photophobia, and the pupil is normal. In acute glaucoma the pupil is dilated and the cornea is hazy.

Posterior uveitis must be differentiated from vitreous hemorrhage where no sign of inflammation is present and the vitreous is filled with red blood cells.

LABORATORY EXAMINATIONS: Extensive laboratory investigations are indicated in an attempt to determine the etiologic basis of the uveitis; however, this is not fruitful in many instances. Blood examinations (CBC, serology), skin tests for tuberculosis, histoplasmosis and toxoplasmosis, and complement fixation tests for toxoplasmosis brucellosis, are among the more common tests. The feces should be examined for parasites.

TREATMENT: Cycloplegics and mydriatics are the more important medications for nonspecific treatment. A cycloplegic immobilizes the iris and the ciliary body and thus quiets the eye and reduces pupillary spasm, the protein content of the aqueous humor, and the pain. Atropine 1% or scopolamine 0.25% solution, 1-3 times daily, should be instilled in the affected eye. Mydriatic drops help to dilate the pupil, reduce the amount of blood in the iris, and prevent posterior synechiae. Phenylephrine hydrochloride 10% (Neosynephrine) drops, a strong mydriatic solution, should be instilled in the affected eye 2-3 times a day.

Corticosteroids are additional nonspecific drugs used in the treatment of uveitis. They can be administered topically (drops or ointment), subconjunctivally, or systemically. If only anterior uveitis is present, corticosteroid drops (Inflamase forte, Prednefrin forte, Decadron) can be instilled several times a day (2-3 times a day) if the case is not severe. If the inflammation is severe the drops can be instilled every hour.

Subconjunctival administration of steroids is very effective; however, it causes local reaction and discomfort. Methylprednisolone acetate (Depo-Medrol) 20-40 mg and triamcinolone acetonide suspension (Kenalog) are the two more common long-acting corticosteroids used for subconjunctival administration. Topical anesthetic drops, Dorsacaine or Ophthetic, should be applied 2-3 times before injecting the corticosteroid. Lidocaine 2% (Xylocaine 2%), 0. 2-0. 3 ml solution, administered together with the corticosteroid, reduces the discomfort of the subconjunctival injection.

The systemic administration of a corticosteroid, 40-120 mg of Prednisone daily, or its equivalent, is advised if the anterior uveitis is very severe or if posterior uveitis is present. Higher doses are indicated only in selected cases.

A few ophthalmologists prefer to start steroid treatment with intravenous ACTH. Forty units of ACTH are dissolved in 500 cc of physiologic solution and given over a period of eight hours.

Other nonspecific drugs such as antimetabolite, typhoid vaccine, salicylates, phenylbutasone, indomethacin, antilymphocyte serum and milk injection are considered to be effective medications in certain cases; however, none of these should be considered as primary treatment on the basis of emergency treatment.

Specific treatments are available for certain types of uveitis. For example, toxoplasmosis may be treated with pyrimethamine (Daraprim) and sulfadiazine. These types of treatment are not considered as emergency situations and, therefore, are not discussed in this book.

D. ENDOPHTHALMITIS
(PANOPHTHALMITIS)

Endophthalmitis is an inflammatory process inside the eye, including vitreous abscess and other infectious or inflammatory processes within the scleral envelope. If the inflammatory process is widespread and all three coats of the eye (sclera, uvea, retina) as well as the vitreous are involved, the condition is called panophthalmitis. Occasionally, the line of demarcation between the two conditions is not too clear.

Intraocular inflammation can be classified as follows:

    A. Exogenous
    B. Endogenous

In most cases of exogenous types of inflammation, the infectious organism has been introduced by a penetrating injury. Endophthalmitis may occur also after surgical procedures of the globe, occasionally many weeks after surgery due to a surgical wound which has not completely healed. Intraocular infection may occur also with corneal ulcer, as an extension of the process into the intraocular tissue. Spread of infection from adjacent tissue (orbit, sinuses) also can cause endophthalmitis (panophthalmitis).

Endogenous endophthalmitis can be caused by metastasis of bacteria, fungus, or parasites from a focus elsewhere in the body. Endophthalmitis can be the result of a blood-borne infection. Necrosis of intraocular tissues often results in severe ocular inflammation resembling endophthalmitis (tumor necrosis).

The common etiologic agents of bacterial infection are:

1. Staphylococci
2. Pneumococci
3. Streptococci
4. Clostridium welchii
5. Bacillus subtilis
6. Pseudomonas aeruginosa

The etiologic agents for micotic infection are:

Actinomyces
Aspergillus
Blastomyces
Candida
Coccidioides
Cryptococcus
Phycomycetes
Sporotrichum

Rarely, rickettsial disease such as epidemic typhus or metazoan infection such as ascariasis (toxocara canis) can be the etiologic agent of endophthalmitis.

SIGNS AND SYMPTOMS: As a general rule, bacterial infection develops fast, while fungus infection progresses slowly, sometimes weeks after injury. The patient with endophthalmitis is uncomfortable. Pain in or around the eye is present in most cases. If the infection is bacterial, occasionally low-grade fever and leucocytosis may be found. The vision is deteriorated to hand movements or light perception in almost all cases. Edema and congestion of the lids are present. Mild protrusion of the globe is not uncommon. Chemosis of the conjunctiva and haziness of the cornea are seen in most cases. Inflammatory cells and purulent exudate may present into and collect in the anterior chamber (hypopyon) (Fig. 3-5). On fundus examination, the red reflex may appear as a greenish color. Details of the retina cannot be seen.

TREATMENT: The treatment of endophthalmitis is disappointing. Early recognition and prompt treatment is necessary to restore useful vision.

Bacterial infection requires massive doses of antibiotics. Three routes -- systemic, subconjunctival, and topical -- of administration of the antibiotic is indicated in all cases. Ampicillin 4.0 gm/day, with chloramphenicol 3.0 gm/day is suggested by many ophthalmologists. Gentamicin (Garamycin) 100 mg per day intramuscularly, or cephalothin (Keflin) or cephaloridine (Loridine) 4.0 gm/day is widely used in cases of endophthalmitis. Tetracyclines seem to be less effective. The intravenous administration of an antibiotic is preferred in bacterial endophthalmitis.

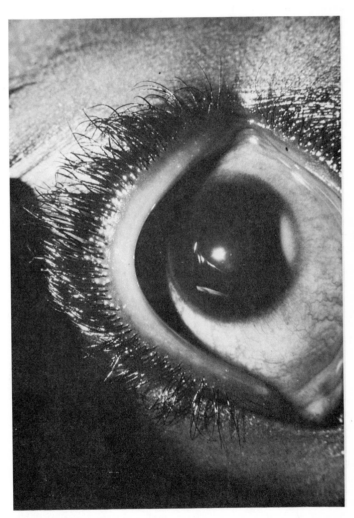

Fig. 3-5. Hypopyon

A synthetic penicillin such as ampicillin 250 mg, methicillin 500 mg, gentamicin 40 mg, cephaloridine 50 mg, and cephalothin 50 mg are the more effective antibiotics for subconjunctival use. Subconjunctival injections may be administered twice a day and should be done only after instillation of a topical anesthetic (2 or 3 times) such as Dorsacaine (benoxinate hydrochloride 0.4%) or Ophthaine (proparacain hydrochloride 0.5%). Lidocaine 2% (Xylocaine 2%) in amounts of 0.2-0.3 cc together with the antibiotic injection, reduces the pain associated with the subconjunctival injection. Topical instillation of other antibiotics such as neomycin, polymyxin, and bacitracin helps in the combined effort to save the globe.

A cycloplegic such as Atropine 1%-2% or Scopolamine 0.25% should also be used three times a day.

Intraocular injection of antibiotics is an ultimate and dangerous procedure in the case of bacterial endophthalmitis. It should not be considered as an emergency procedure. If it is indicated it has to be performed by an experienced ophthalmic surgeon.

The use of steroids with antibiotics is advised by many ophthalmologists. The rationale of this therapy is that steroids reduce the massive inflammatory response of the eye, that is, in itself, very destructive. Opponents of this combined therapy emphasize the possibility of spreading the causative organism, especially if it is not responsive to the antibiotics used.

Fungal endophthalmitis should be treated with amphotericin B and nystatin. One hundred and fifty micrograms of amphotericin B in 0.5 ml of sterile water can be injected subconjunctivally once or twice a day. Amphotericin B eyedrops 10 mg/cc should be instilled into the conjunctival sac every hour. Systemic or intraocular administration of amphotericin B should be considered only in selected cases because of the high toxicity of the drug and because of the low penetration into the eye. The drug is given intravenously. The initial dose is 0.05-0.1 mg/kg of body weight. This amount should be administered by slow infusion over a period of six hours. The amount of amphotericin B should be increased by 0.1 mg/kg of body weight on consecutive or alternate days until the maximal dose of 1.0 mg/kg of body weight is reached. This treatment must be continued until there is a response or until there are signs of renal toxicity.

Nystatin is a very insoluble drug. A special diluent supplied by Squibb may be used to dissolve 200,000 units. This suspension can be used for topical instillation or subconjunctival injection. The absorption of the latter is extremely poor. Systemic administration of Nystatin (2 gm/day) has very little effect in fungus endophthalmitis. Flucytosine 200 mg/kg/day has a better result in Candida endophthalmitis.

There is no effective medication against endophthalmitis caused by rickettsia or metazoan infection.

The concept of antibiotic potentiation of ocular fungus infection has not been clearly established. Because of the diagnostic difficulty in distinguishing between bacterial and fungal intraocular infection and the much more common incidence of bacterial infection, it is believed that withholding antibiotic therapy is not in the best interest of the patient. In doubtful cases, the possibility of successfully treating bacterial infection is much greater than treating fungal infection and, therefore, antibiotic therapy is recommended.

Corticosteroid therapy promotes ocular fungus infection. Therefore, its use is not recommended if the etiology of endophthalmitis is in doubt.

PROGNOSIS: Endophthalmitis and panophthalmitis have poor prognoses, especially if the etiologic agent is fungal, rickettsial, or parasitic. If endophthalmitis is caused by bacteria, the eye can be saved by early diagnosis and prompt treatment with antibiotics. However, very often the final result concerning visual acuity is disappointing.

FREQUENTLY USED ANTIBACTERIALS**

Drug	Dose	Spectrum	Side Effects
Penicillin G.	200,000 to 400,000 U. q. 4 to 6 hrs. (o.) : 300,000 U. q. 4 to 6 hrs. (i.m); may go as high as 20,000,000 U./d.	Gm+ cocci and bacilli; Gm– cocci; spirochetes.	Hypersensitivity–usually rash and/or fever, occasionally serum sickness; less commonly anaphylactoid reactions; generally safest of all antibiotics.
Penicillin V (V–Cillin, Pen–Vee); semisynthetic penicillin.	250 mg. q. i. d.	Gm+ cocci and bacilli; Gm– cocci; less effective than penicillin G but more stable in acid of the stomach.	Hypersensitivity as with penicillin G.
Phenethicillin (Syncillin, Chemipen, Maxipen); semisynthetic penicillin.	125 to 250 mg t. i. d.	Gm+ cocci and bacilli; Gm– cocci; less effective than penicillin G, but more stable in acid of the stomach.	Hypersensitivity as with penicillin G.
Ampicillin (Polycillin, Penbritin); semisynthetic penicillin.	500 to 1000 mg. q. 6 hrs. (o); 500 mg. q. 6 hrs. (i. m.)	Gm+ organisms sensitive to penicillin G as well as a variety of Gm– rods; e. g., H. influenza, E. coli, S. typhosa, etc. Used for therapy of intraocular spirochetes.	Hypersensitivity as with penicillin G; elevation of SGOT.

Drug	Dose	Uses	Toxicity
Cloxacillin (Tegopen, Orbenin); semisynthetic penicillin.	500 to 1000 mg. q. 4 to 6 hrs. (o.) 1000 mg. q. 4 to 6 hrs. (i. m.)	Penicillin G resistant staphylococci.	Hypersensitivity as with penicillin G.
Methicillin (Staphcillin, Dimocillin); semisynthetic penicillin.	1 to 2 gm. q. 4 to 6 hrs. (i. m.)	Penicillin G resistant staphylococci.	Hypersensitivity, as with penicillin G; leukopenia, neutropenia, nephritis, superinfections with Gm– bacteria.
Nafcillin (Unipen); semisynthetic penicillin.	500 to 1000 mg. q. 4 to 6 hrs. (o.) 500 to 1000 mg. q. 4 to 6 hrs. (i. m.)	Penicillin G resistant staphylococci.	Hypersensitivity as with penicillin G.
Oxacillin (Resistopen, Prostaphlin); semisynthetic penicillin.	500 to 1000 mg. q. 4 to 6 hrs. (o.) or (i. m.)	Penicillin G resistant staphylococci.	Hypersensitivity as with penicillin G; gastrointestinal complaints, anorexia, nausea, etc.; elevation of SGOT.
Tetracyclines: chlortetracycline* (Aureomycin), oxytetracycline* (Terramycin), tetracycline* (Achromycin); Demethylchlortetracycline (Declomycin).	250 to 500 mg. q. i. d. (o.) 150 to 225 q. i. d. (o.)	Gm+ cocci, Gm– bacilli and cocci; rickettsia, psittacosis and lymphogranuloma group viruses.	Gastrointestinal disturbances, hepatic toxicity (during pregnancy), renal toxicity from outdated drug (Fanconi-like syndrome), mucous membrane toxicity, discoloration of teeth in children, superinfections.

FREQUENTLY USED ANTIBACTERIALS**

Drug	Dose	Spectrum	Side Effects
Streptomycin	250 to 500 mg. q. i. d. (i. m.)	Gm− organisms and tubercle bacilli, occasionally Gm+; resistance development is rapid; usually used in combination with another antibiotic.	Vestibular damage, dose-related deafness is seen rarely; hypersensitivity usually is manifest as a rash, occasionally urticaria, angioneurotic edema, or exfoliative dermatitis; eosinophilia with long-term therapy.
Chloramphenicol* (Chloromycetin).	250 to 500 mg. q. 6 hrs. (o.); also available (i. m.) and (i. v.)	Gm−bacilli (Proteus and Pseudomonas may be resistant), rickettsia, moderately effective against Gm+ cocci and bacilli, and Gm− cocci.	Gastrointestinal upsets, hematopoietic depression, "Gray syndrome" in the newborn, superinfections, especially Monilia.
Neomycin*	8 to 16 gm. for 1 to 2 d. (o.) to prepare for bowel surgery; 10 to 15 mg./kg. per day (i. m.) rarely used.	Similar to streptomycin; not effective against Pseudomonas.	Parenterally; ototoxicity and nephrotoxicity; low incidence of allergic skin reactions with topical use.

Drug	Dosage	Organisms	Adverse Effects
Polymyxin B* (Aerosporin).	For Pseudomonas especially; (i. m.) or (i. v.) up to 2.5 mg./kg. daily.	Most Gm− organisms, especially Pseudomonas.	Nephrotoxicity, mild neurotoxicity.
Kanamycin (Kantrex).	7.5 to 15 mg./kg. daily (i. m.) or (i. v.); 1 gm. q. 4 hrs. (o.) to prepare for bowel surgery.	Similar to neomycin.	Similar to neomycin.
Bacitracin*	Not absorbed (o.); rarely used (i. m.)	Gm+ cocci and bacilli.	Nephrotoxicity with parenteral use.
Colistin* (Colymycin).	2.5 to 5 mg./kg (i. m.) daily.	Gm− organisms, especially Pseudomonas (not Proteus).	Nephrotoxicity; mild neurotoxicity.
Erythromycin* (Erythrocin, Ilotycin, Ilosone).	250 to 500 mg. q. 6 hrs. (o.)	Gm+ cocci and bacilli; Neisseria and Spirochetes.	Adverse effects are rare; cholestatic hepatitis with estolate salt (Ilosone).
Novobiocin (Albamycin, Cathomycin).	250 to 500 mg. q. 6 hrs. (o.); rarely used.	Staphylococci, Pneumococci, Clostridia, Neisseria, H. influenza, and some Proteus.	Skin eruptions, fever, jaundice, and gastrointestinal disturbances.
Ristocetin (Spontin).	25 mg./kg. per day (i. v.); rarely used.	Gm+ cocci and bacilli (includes penicillin resistant staphylococci, tubercle bacilli.	Phlebitis, fever, skin eruptions, thrombocytopenia, bone marrow depression.

FREQUENTLY USED ANTIBACTERIALS**

Drug	Dose	Spectrum	Side Effects
Vancomycin (Vancocin).	2 to 4 gm. daily (i.v.); rarely used.	Gm+ cocci and bacilli (includes penicillin resistant staphylococci).	Phlebitis, fever, skin eruptions, nephrotoxicity, ototoxicity.
Oleandomycin (Matromycin); triacetyloleandomycin (Cyclamycin. TAO).	250 to 500 mg. q. 6 hrs. (o.)	Gm+ cocci and bacilli; Neisseria and H. influenza.	Cholestatic hepatitis (triacetyloleandomycin); gastrointestinal disturbances.
Cephalothin (Keflin).	500 to 1000 mg. q. 6 hrs. (i.m.) or (i.v.)	Gm+ cocci (includes penicillin resistant staphylococci), Gm− cocci and bacilli, except Proteus and Pseudomonas.	Pain, phlebitis, drug rash, reversible neutropenia.
Lincomycin (Lincocin).	500 to 1000 mg. q. 6 hrs. (o.); 500 mg. q. 12 hrs. (i.m.) or (i.v.)	Gm+ cocci (including penicillin resistant staphylococci) except S. faecalis.	Diarrhea, pruritus vulvae and ani, abnormalities of liver function, superinfections.
Gentamycin* (Garamycin).	0.4 mg./kg. q. 6 hrs. (i.m.)	Gm+ cocci, Gm− bacilli, including Pseudomonas.	Vestibular toxicity, nephrotoxicity, phototoxicity.

Sulfonamides: sulfisoxazole* (Gantrisin); sulfamethoxypyridazine (Kynex); sulfisomidine (Elkosin); sulfadimethoxine (Madribon); sulfacetamide* (Sulamyd): triple sulfa: sulfadiazine, sulfamerazine, sulfamethazine.	Usually 1 to 2 gm. to start, then 1 gm. q. 6 hrs.	Gm+ cocci and bacilli; Gm– cocci and some bacilli; psittacosis and lymphogranuloma group viruses, especially trachoma.	Crystalluria, hypersensitivity reactions including Stevens-Johnson syndrome, blood dyscrasias.

* Commonly used topically. (o.)=orally.

** Reprinted by permission of the author and the publisher: Scheie, H. G. and Albert, D. M. : Adler's Textbook, Philadelphia, London, Toronto, W. B. Saunders Co., Copyright (C) 1969.

BIBLIOGRAPHY

1. Burns, R. P. : Eyelids, lacrimal apparatus and conjunctiva. Ann Rev Arch Ophthal 79:211, 1968.

2. Coles, R. S. : Steroid therapy in uveitis. Int Ophthal Clin 6:869, 1966.

3. Ellis, P. P. and Smith, P. L. : Ocular Therapeutics and Pharmacology. Mosby, St. Louis, 1969.

4. Hertzberg, R. : Exogenous mycotic endophthalmitis following cataract extraction. Aust J Ophthal 2:84, 1974.

5. Infectious Diseases of the Conjunctiva and Cornea. Symposium of the New Orleans Academy of Ophthalmology. Mosby, St. Louis, 1963.

6. Jones, D. B. : Early diagnosis and therapy of bacterial corneal ulcers. Int Ophthal Clin 14:1, 1973.

7. Jones, D. B. : The early diagnosis and management of bacterial endophthalmitis. In: Ocular Inflammatory Disease. Golden, B. (Ed.) Charles C. Thomas Co. , Springfield, Ill. , 1974.

8. Jones, L. T. : The lacrimal secretory system and its treatment. Am J Ophthal 62:47, 1966.

9. Kaufman, H. E. : Chemotherapy of herpes simplex keratitis. Invest Ophthal 2:504, 1963.

10. Kaufman, H. E. : The uvea. Ann Rev Arch Ophthal 75:407, 1967.

11. Leopold, I. H. : Drug therapy in uveitis. Am J Ophthal 56:709, 1963.

12. Leopold, I. H. : Problems in the use of antibiotics in ophthalmology. Leopold, I. H. editor: Symposium on Ocular Therapy, Vol. 3, Mosby, St. Louis, 1968.

13. Peyman, G. A. and Herbst, R. : Bacterial endophthalmitis treatment with intraocular injection of gentamicin and dexamethasone. Arch Ophthal 91:46, 1974.

14. Records, R. E. : The cephalosporins in ophthalmology. Surv Ophthal 13:345, 1969.

15. Records, R. E. : The penicillins in ophthalmology. Surv Ophthal 13:207, 1969.

16. Robertson, D. M. , Riley, F. C. and Hermans, P. E. : Endogenous Candida oculomycosis. Report of two patients treated with flucytosine. Arch Ophthal 9:33, 1974.

17. Suie, T. and Havener, W. H. : Mycology of the eye: A review. Am J Ophthal 56:63, 1963.

18. Suie, T. : Microbiology of the Eye. Am Acad Ophthal Otolaryng, Rochester, 1964.

19. Vaughan, D. G. Jr. : Corneal ulcers. Surv Ophthal 3:203, 1958.

20. Woods, A. C. : Endogenous Inflammation of the Uveal Tract. The Williams and Wilkins Co. , Baltimore, 1961.

CHAPTER 4

GLAUCOMA

Glaucoma is still a common cause of blindness throughout the world. Every physician should be aware of glaucoma and must understand some of the present day concepts. A physician should know its symptoms and be constantly alert for its possible presence.

The eye has its optimal tension; it is called the intraocular pressure. In normal conditions the pressure is 14-20 mm Hg. When the intraocular pressure increases to a dangerously high level the condition is known as glaucoma. The condition might be compared to an overly inflated ball in which pressure is transmitted equally to all points of the inner aspect (the coat) of the ball. In the eye, this coat is the sclera. The area where the optic nerve enters the eye is weaker than the rest of the coat and thus the optic nerve is highly vulnerable to damage by increased intraocular pressure.

Elevated intraocular pressure could result from an increased rate of formation of aqueous humor, from an increased resistance to outflow of the aqueous from the eye, or from some mechanical block of the aqueous flow on its route from the ciliary body to the periphery of the anterior chamber.

Today, blindness from glaucoma can be prevented by early recognition of the disease and proper treatment.

The literature on the theoretical and investigative aspects of glaucoma is extensive. Since the primary interest of this manual is to deal with emergency and urgent ophthalmologic conditions, these aspects of the disease are not discussed in this book.

CLASSIFICATION: Glaucoma can be divided into two major groups:

1. Primary glaucoma
2. Secondary glaucoma

Primary glaucoma implies a separate disease unrelated to any other ocular or general condition.

Secondary glaucoma is a consequence of another recognizable ocular or orbital disease.

Primary glaucoma can be further classified as follows:

A. Glaucoma of the adult
B. Glaucoma of the infant and juvenile

The adult type of glaucoma is divided into:

1. Simple glaucoma (chronic simple glaucoma, open-angle glaucoma

2. Closed-angle glaucoma (narrow-angle glaucoma, angle-closure glaucoma)

At the symposium on glaucoma organized by the Council for International Organization of Medical Sciences in 1954, the terms simple glaucoma and closed-angle glaucoma were chosen to designate the primary glaucomas. However, in the United States, the terms mentioned in the brackets above are commonly used.

Congenital glaucoma of the infantile type is manifested during the first three years of life. This condition is rare. It is believed that most of these glaucomas are hereditary.

Glaucoma is classified as "juvenile" when it occurs between the ages of three and 35. This type of glaucoma is relatively uncommon.

The prevalence of glaucoma in the general population over age 40 is about 2%. Primary glaucoma can occur at any age; adult glaucoma occurs in individuals over 35 years of age.

Simple glaucoma occurs much more frequently than angle-closure glaucoma. Acute glaucoma comprises less than 10% of primary glaucoma cases. However, from the viewpoint of the emergency room physician, acute glaucoma is the most important type and the most likely to be encountered in ophthalmologic emergencies.

Our present classification of primary glaucoma into two main groups (chronic simple glaucoma and angle-closure glaucoma) originates from gonioscopic and tonographic studies of the aqueous outflow. Gonioscopy is the visualization of the angle of the anterior chamber and the trabecula. In the case of chronic simple glaucoma, the angle is widely open. Thus, the previous name of this group of glaucoma was open-angle glaucoma (Fig. 4-1).

Closed-angle glaucoma is characterized by a very narrow or closed angle. This condition is associated with episodes of high intraocular pressure (Fig. 4-2).

Secondary glaucoma can be caused by many ocular conditions such as:

1. Corneal lesions with iris adherence (also called corneal adherent leucoma)
2. Uveal tract changes
   a. Anterior and/or posterior uveitis
   b. Tumor in the choroid, ciliary body, or iris
   c. Essential iris atrophy
3. Pathologic lens conditions
   a. Subluxation of the lens
   b. Dislocation of the lens
   c. Intumescence of the lens
   d. Phacotoxic or phacoanaphylactic reaction due to a cataractous lens

4. Trauma
   a. Hemorrhage into the anterior or posterior chamber or into the vitreous body
   b. Angle recess
   c. Hemolytic
5. Vascular conditions
   a. Central retinal vein occlusion
   b. Central retinal artery occlusion
   c. Rubeosis iridis (Neovascular glaucoma)
6. Associated with use of drugs (corticosteroid induced glaucoma - topical or systemic -)
7. Orbital conditions
   a. Tumor
   b. Inflammation
   c. Pulsating vascular lesions (carotic cavernous fistula)
8. Following intraocular surgery, or traumatic (perforating) injury
   a. Epithelial ingrowth
   b. Failure of reformation of the anterior chamber after intraocular surgery, and occlusion of the chamber angle

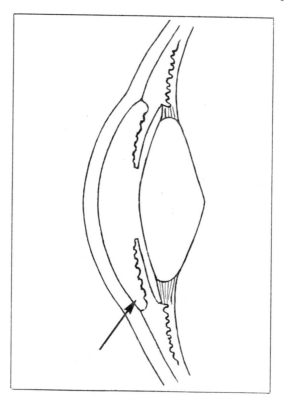

Fig. 4-1. Deep anterior chamber found in chronic simple glaucoma

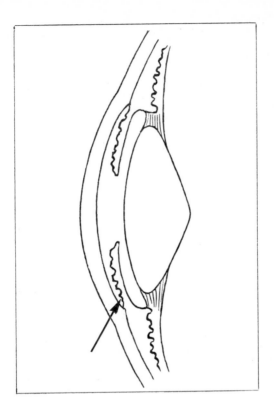

Fig. 4-2. Shallow anterior chamber found in narrow (closed) angle glaucoma

Absolute glaucoma, or fere absolute glaucoma are terms concerning glaucomatous conditions. An eye which is blind as a result of glaucoma, regardless of the type, is called absolute glaucoma. An eye with very little residual vision (light perception or hand movements) caused by glaucoma is called fere absolute glaucoma.

PHYSIOLOGIC ASPECTS OF GLAUCOMA: The intraocular pressure is determined by: a) the rate of aqueous production of the ciliary body, b) the resistance to the outflow of aqueous humor from the eye.

The exact mechanism of aqueous production is not completely understood. It is most certain that the central nervous system influences aqueous production and the resistance to outflow. It is assumed that electrolytes, water, protein, and other components of the aqueous humor are produced through diffusion, ultrafiltration, and secretion, by the ciliary body and the ciliary process.

From the ciliary body and the ciliary processes the aqueous humor enters into the posterior chamber. The fluid passes through the pupil into the anterior chamber. The aqueous humor leaves the anterior chamber through the trabecular meshwork and enters Schlemm's canal. Efferent channels conduct the fluid from Schlemm's canal to the venous system.

In simple glaucoma the angle is open and it is believed that the cause of the elevated intraocular pressure is the increased resistance to aqueous humor outflow. Hypersecretion is a relatively rare cause of glaucoma.

Angle-closure glaucoma or closed-angle glaucoma occurs in an eye with a very narrow anterior chamber angle. When the pupil is dilated or the iris contracts, the root of the iris may obstruct the anterior chamber angle and this mechanical effect impairs the outflow of the aqueous humor.

We assume that infantile glaucoma is a result of an imperfectly developed drainage mechanism. It is believed that incomplete cleavage of the periphery of the uveal tract from the corneoscleral wall is the cause of this congenital disease.

Juvenile glaucoma also results from a faulty drainage mechanism. The course is similar to that of simple glaucoma, except that it is more severe in the juvenile age group.

The most important mechanism in secondary glaucoma is the increased resistance to aqueous outflow in the trabecular meshwork, the canal of Schlemm, or, occasionally, the aqueous veins. Inflammatory adhesions between the iris and the lens also block the normal flow of aqueous from the posterior chamber to the anterior chamber and cause elevated intraocular pressure. Various inflammatory cells, red blood cells, protein, lens debris, and pigment can obstruct the trabecular meshwork and, in this way, cause elevated intraocular pressure. Trauma may cause injury to the trabecula (for example, atrophy, hyalinization) and be responsible for faulty aqueous outflow. The exact mechanism of elevated intraocular pressure in the case of an intraocular tumor is not well understood. The space occupied by the tumor, toxic products of the tumor, and mechanical angle closure by pushing the iris forward, are all considered to cause secondary glaucoma.

In conclusion, secondary glaucoma is the state of elevated intraocular pressure associated with other ocular disease which interferes with the normal physiologic circulation of the aqueous humor.

SIGNS AND SYMPTOMS

INFANTILE GLAUCOMA: The classical triad of photophobia, blepharospasm, and tearing are the more common initial signs of infantile glaucoma. Unexplained photophobia or tearing are important signs of the disease and should not be overlooked by the physician. Corneal haze may or may not be present in the initial phase of the disease. Enlargement of the cornea or enlargement of the

entire eyeball is almost always a diagnostic sign of infantile glaucoma. If the corneal diameter is larger than 12 mm, the physician
should be suspicious of glaucoma. In these cases, the intraocular
pressure is almost always elevated. In general, accurate tonometry cannot be performed in the emergency room. Without general
anesthesia and complete rest one cannot achieve accurate measurements of the intraocular pressure of a child.

SIMPLE GLAUCOMA: Simple glaucoma causes no early symptoms.
Occasionally, the patient may present with dull headache when the
pressure is high. When the intraocular pressure is very high and
the corneal epithelium is edematous, blurred vision or a rainbow
effect around lights may occur. In general, visual acuity is not effected until late in the course of the disease. Tonometry reveals
increased intraocular pressure. External examination does not reveal any abnormality. Ophthalmoscopic examination may be normal
in the early stage of simple glaucoma. Later, the temporal disc
margin thins and glaucomatous cupping becomes wider and deeper.
The vessels are displaced nasally. At this stage, various visual
field defects can be observed. One should remember that this type
of glaucoma rarely appears in the emergency room and simple glaucoma (open-angle glaucoma) is not a disease of real emergency.

ANGLE-CLOSURE GLAUCOMA (CLOSED-ANGLE GLAUCOMA): An
acute attack of closed-angle glaucoma is characterized by severe
pain in or around the eye. The vision is blurred. Gastrointestinal
symptoms such as nausea and vomiting are often present and sometimes mask the disease.

The intraocular pressure is elevated and the cornea is edematous.
The pupil is moderately dilated and reacts poorly, or not at all, to
stimulus. The anterior chamber is very shallow. On external examination, chemosis of the conjunctiva and ciliary injection are
found. Details of the fundus cannot be seen because of the edema of
the cornea.

Angle-closure glaucoma does not always appear with all the above-
mentioned classical signs and symptoms of the disease. Sometimes
the history of pain and blurred vision only suggest the diagnosis.
Occasionally, the so-called "preglaucomal or interval glaucoma"
conditions may exist. Intraocular pressure may be normal or slightly elevated between mild attacks which have been provoked by pupillary dilatation (being in darkness for a long period of time). The
physician must be aware of these conditions and must know that a
"real" acute attack may occur by pupillary dilatation at any time.

DIFFERENTIAL DIAGNOSIS OF GLAUCOMA
(Special emphasis on acute attack)

As mentioned above, simple glaucoma or infantile glaucoma is
rarely presented in the emergency room. If, on occasion, such a
case is encountered and the diagnosis of glaucoma is suspected,
there is always enough time to refer the patient to the ophthalmolo-

gist for further evaluation. Therefore, the differential diagnosis is not discussed in this framework.

The following must be considered in the differential diagnosis of an acute attack of glaucoma: a) acute iritis, b) acute iridocyclitis, c) acute conjunctivitis.

In acute iritis or iridocyclitis, the pupil is constricted (not dilated), the photophobia is more pronounced, and the pain is less severe than in acute glaucoma. In acute conjunctivitis there is little or no pain, the visual acuity is unchanged, and the pupil reacts to stimulus.

Acute glaucoma can be easily overlooked when the gastrointestinal symptoms of glaucoma are very severe and mimic an acute abdominal condition. The same is true in the case of a patient with an abdominal condition which was treated with atropine or atropine-like medication and the systemic medication precipitates the acute attack of glaucoma. An eye having a narrow angle and treated for any reason with mydriatics or cycloplegics also can develop an acute attack as a result of the medication.

EMERGENCY TREATMENT

Emergency treatment is indicated only in an acute attack of angle-closure glaucoma (closed-angle glaucoma) or a severe case of secondary glaucoma. Medical therapy should be administered whenever possible.

Therapy consists of:

A. Topical treatment with parasympathomimetic cholinergic agents or anticholinesterase drugs
B. Systemic treatment with carbonic anhydrase inhibitors or hyperosmotic agents, or both

A. TOPICAL TREATMENT: Pilocarpine, 2%, eyedrops are used as soon as the diagnosis is established. The drops can be instilled every 10 minutes. Eserine, 0.75%, eyedrops also can be used at the same time intervals. Miotic agents retract the iris from the corneoscleral wall and reopen the anterior chamber angle. This allows the aqueous to leave the eye through the physiologic route.

If the acute attack has been present for a few hours, the iris muscle may not respond to miotic drops and the pupil will remain dilated.

A strong miotic such as isofluophate (DFP) or echothiophate (Phospholine iodide), strong anticholinesterase drugs, cause congestion of the iris stroma and the ciliary body and, therefore, should be avoided. For this reason, in an acute attack many ophthalmologists do not use pilocarpine in concentrations higher than 2%, or eserine higher than 1%.

B. SYSTEMIC TREATMENT: Often, the patient suffering from an acute attack of glaucoma is nauseous. Therefore, the intravenous route of medication is desirable.

Acetazolamide (DIAMOX), 500 mg I. V. , should first be administered. This medication should be continued with a dose of 250 mg every four hours by mouth after the nausea has subsided. Practically, there is no known contraindication to this kind of medication except proved hypersensitivity to the drug. Diamox is a carbonic anhydrase inhibitor. Diamox reduces the production of the aqueous humor and in that way reduces also the elevated intraocular pressure. Other carbonic anhydrase inhibitors such as methazolamide (Neptazane) and dichlorphenamide (Daramide) are rarely used, if at all, in case of an acute attack.

MANNITOL is a hyperosmotic agent. Mannitol is administered intravenously in amounts of 1. 5-2. 0 gm/kg body weight in 20% solution. Before the start of this treatment the physician should check the patient's heart condition to determine whether he can tolerate the required amount of medication. The total amount of mannitol is given during a one-hour period. Prior to administration the mannitol solution should be checked for the presence of crystals. If crystals are present, warming the bottle containing the solution will eliminate the crystals in the fluid. Mannitol is not metabolized in a significant amount and, therefore, it can be used safely in the presence of diabetes.

UREA (Urevert) is another hyperosmotic agent. It also is administered by intravenous route in amounts of 1 gm/kg body weight. This medication is extremely effective; however, its use is contraindicated in patients suffering from liver or kidney disorders.

GLYCEROL is one of the more commonly used hyperosmotic agents. It is administered by mouth. It is safe and it can be given even in the ophthalmologist's office. The usual amount is 1 ml/kg body weight in 50% solution. Its main advantage is its easy use. However, if the patient is nauseous or vomiting, often he will not tolerate glycerol. Glycerol is metabolized as a carbohydrate and so may cause hyperglycemia and glycosuria. If it is administered intravenously, in error, it can cause hematuria by damaging the afferent glomerular arterioles.

The combination of miotics, carbonic anhydrase inhibitor, and hyperosmotic agent is the best and most effective combined medication to treat an acute attack of glaucoma. After intensive treatment, the intraocular pressure will usually fall to normal level within 30 minutes to a few hours. The visual acuity improves gradually. Miotic drops such as pilocarpine should be continued every four hours. Miotics also should be instilled in the fellow eye to avoid the danger of an acute attack in that eye.

FINAL TREATMENT: Acute attack of closed-angle glaucoma almost certainly will reoccur if the eye is not operated on. Therefore, after successful treatment of the first acute attack of glaucoma, the patient's eyes should be examined and evaluated by an ophthalmologist. Gonioscopy and tonography should be performed. Surgical treatment (peripheral iridectomy) should be done as soon as the condition of the eye is suitable for surgery.

TREATMENT OF SECONDARY GLAUCOMA

In general, the patient appears in the emergency room with this type of glaucoma because of severe pain or the previously mentioned signs of an acute attack of glaucoma, namely, nausea, vomiting, and blurred vision.

The treatment of secondary glaucoma is almost as varied as the cases. Thus, the treatment must be divided into two main groups:

A. Treatment of the underlying disease
B. Treatment of the elevated intraocular pressure

The emergency room physician must concentrate his efforts to relieve the acute symptoms and to reduce the patient's discomfort.

To reduce intraocular pressure, carbonic anhydrase inhibitors and hyperosmotic agents are safe and helpful drugs. In certain cases, sympathomimetic eyedrops such as Neosynephrine 10% can be used to reduce aqueous humor production and, in that way, also the intraocular pressure.

Five hundred mg of Diamox are administered intravenously. Intravenous administration of the drug provides quick action. Diamox should be continued in a dose of 250 mg four times a day by mouth. Mannitol, urea, or glycerol could be added. The dosage and the contraindications for treatment of an attack of secondary glaucoma are the same as those mentioned previously for acute closed-angle glaucoma. It is advisable not to administer pilocarpine drops unless the etiology of the secondary glaucoma is clear. Pilocarpine causes vasocongestion and might worsen the condition of the underlying disease responsible for the elevated intraocular pressure. The patient might benefit with local treatment of epinephrine, norepinephrine 1% eyedrops (Eppy, Glaucon) or Neosynephrine 10% twice a day.

FINAL TREATMENT: As mentioned previously, the type of treatment varies according to the etiology of the secondary glaucoma. The glaucoma that accompanies some inflammations of the eye, such as iritis and iridocyclitis, may benefit quickly from corticosteroids and cycloplegic eyedrops. Others, such as pupillary block, need surgical intervention (iridectomy) to provide prompt relief. Glaucomas that develop due to closure of main blood vessels of the eye can be quite resistant to treatment and sometimes the decision is difficult as to whether to be conservative or to operate on the eye. One principle must be remembered by the physician seeing and treating the patient with a secondary glaucoma: administration of different kinds of medication, except those reducing the intraocular pressure (Diamox, glycerol), should not be done until the proper diagnosis has been established.

BIBLIOGRAPHY

1. Becker, B. and Shaffer, R. N. : Diagnosis and Therapy of the Glaucomas. The C. V. Mosby Co. , St. Louis, 1965.

2. Ferrer, O. M. (ed.): Symposium on Glaucoma. Charles C Thomas, Springfield, 1976.

3. Newell, F. W. (ed.): Glaucoma. Transactions of the First, Second, Third, Fourth, and Fifth Conferences. Josiah Macy, Jr. Foundation, New York, 1956-1960.

4. Scheie, H. G. and Albert, D. M. : Adler's Textbook of Ophthalmology. W. B. Saunders Co. , Philadelphia, London, Toronto, 1969.

5. Symposium on Glaucoma: Tr New Orleans Acad Ophth. The C. V. Mosby Co. , St. Louis, 1967.

CHAPTER 5

TRAUMA: PART I

NONPENETRATING AND NONPERFORATING INJURIES OF THE EYEBALL

Trauma of the eyeball is relatively common despite the well-developed protective mechanism of the visual system. The bony orbital rim prevents many injuries of the eyeball itself. The eyelashes and eyelids are highly sensitive and the lids quickly close reflexively through stimuli. In this way, serious injury to the globe is prevented. The upward rotation of the eye due to a sudden stimulus is an additional reflexive action which protects the cornea from injury.

It should be understood that in many cases the eye might have useful vision if careful attention were provided immediately after the injury. Therefore, the emergency room physician should be familiar with the treatment of a traumatized eye. An ocular injury requires immediate attention, diagnosis, and definitive treatment. Very often, proper first-aid attention can prevent future complications and further deterioration of the condition of the eye. Improper handling and poor management can destroy an injured eye and can cause permanent blindness.

Ocular injuries can be divided into two groups: nonpenetrating injuries, and penetrating and perforating injuries of the eyeball.

NONPENETRATING AND NONPERFORATING INJURIES

Nonpenetrating injuries include:

1. Superficial injuries of the cornea (abrasion, foreign body)
2. Chemical and physical injuries
3. Contusion and concussion injury of the eyeball

1. SUPERFICIAL CORNEAL INJURIES

A. Abrasion of the Cornea

Traumatic removal of the corneal epithelium is called abrasion of the cornea. This condition is not necessarily due to friction from a foreign body in the conjunctival sac or on the cornea. Young mothers suffer from corneal erosion very often because the baby scratches their eyes. Flying objects may injure the corneal epithelium without adhering to the cornea. A corneal abrasion is not a serious condition.

SIGNS AND SYMPTOMS: The patient may complain of foreign-body sensation. Abrasion may cause severe pain. Lacrimation, blepharospasm, and blinking of the eyelid also are common signs of corneal abrasion. Occasionally, photophobia may occur and the conjunctiva is hyperemic. Visual acuity may be normal or only slightly deteriorated.

Examination of the cornea by direct bright light may be negative. The epithelial injury or denudation of the cornea is easily seen when fluorescein dye is instilled into the conjunctival sac. Occasionally, the examination of an eye so injured is difficult. In order to facilitate the examination, the pain associated with the abrasion can be relieved by instillation of local anesthetic eyedrops such as 0.4%-1% benoxinate hydrochloride (Dorsacain) or proparacaine hydrochloride 0.5% (Ophthaine).

Instillation of local anesthetic should not be continued since it delays the re-epithelization of the cornea and masks the diagnosis of possible complications such as infection or anterior uveitis which might cause continuous pain.

TREATMENT: Any debris present in the conjunctival sac should be removed. Administration of a short-acting cycloplegic such as tropicamide 1% (Mydriacyl) or cyclopentolate 0.5% (Cyclogyl) eyedrops is advisable. This will make the eye more comfortable and will reduce secondary iridocyclitis. A broad-spectrum antibiotic such as chloromycetin 1%, drops or ointment, will prevent potential bacterial infection. An eye patch is applied with gentle pressure for one or two days. Corneal abrasion heals relatively quickly, usually within one to three days; however, daily examination is required. If Bowman's membrane is not damaged, no sign of corneal abrasion will remain after injury.

B. Superficial Foreign Bodies

A foreign body such as a glass, wood, or metallic particle may be propelled into the eye by moving machinery (Fig. 5-1). A foreign body also may drop into the eye, or the wind may blow it on the cornea. Multiple foreign bodies may be driven into the cornea by an explosion. The retention of a foreign body on the surface of the eye is the most common ocular injury caused by accident. Organized material causes considerable irritation. A foreign body such as grain may excite an irritative inflammatory reaction with edema and discharge. On the other hand, glass, plastic, or stone may be seen on the cornea without significant reaction.

SIGNS AND SYMPTOMS: The patient suffers from pain, lacrimation, and foreign-body sensation. Repeated blinking may be observed and the visual acuity is reduced. The conjunctiva is hyperemic. If the foreign body has been in the cornea for a long period of time, photophobia may be present. Examination of the cornea, using an oblique moving bright light, may reveal the foreign body. A metallic foreign body is surrounded by a rust ring within a relatively short period of time.

TREATMENT: Administration of topical anesthesia is necessary for removal of a foreign body imbedded in the cornea. Proparacaine,

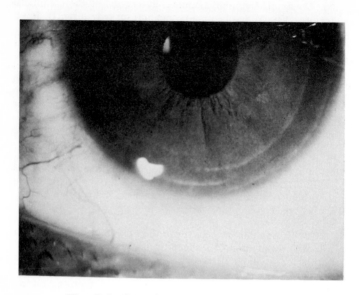

Fig. 5-1. Superficial corneal foreign body

0. 5%-1% (Ophthaine), or tetracain (Pontocaine) eyedrops instilled three to four times into the conjunctival sac provide adequate anesthesia. Removal of a foreign body is best accomplished with a small, sharp instrument. A sterile hypodermic needle is as satisfactory an instrument as is a special foreign body removal spud. The average superficial particle can be dislodged easily with only minimal damage to the surrounding tissue. One must remember that the cornea is thin (less than 1 mm) and, therefore, care must be taken not to perforate it. A cotton-wool applicator is an unsatisfactory instrument for this purpose. It causes extensive damage to the surrounding epithelium and is not suitable to remove rust rings around a metallic foreign body. An unremoved rust ring behaves as an unremoved foreign body and continues to irritate the eye. Therefore, both the foreign body and the rust ring must be removed.

After removal of the foreign body, a short-acting cycloplegic such as tropicamide, 1% (Mydriacyl), or cyclopentolate, 0. 5% (Cyclogyl), eyedrops will reduce the effects of secondary iritis. A broadspectrum antibiotic ointment such as 1% chloromycetin or gentamicin should be used and an eye patch should be applied with gentle pressure for one to several days.

Daily examination of the injured eye and application of an antibiotic and a cycloplegic should be continued until the corneal wound is completely healed. Many ophthalmologists do not patch an eye after removal of a foreign body because patching encourages infection. However, the patient feels more comfortable with a pressure-patch and, therefore, patching is advisable for a few days. Many ophthalmologists use antibiotic drops only, since ointments delay wound healing. However, antibiotic ointments give better protection against infection since it remains in the conjunctival sac for a longer period of time and, therefore, its use is recommended.

To summarize the treatment, in steps:

1. Remove the foreign body (including the rust ring)
2. Administer a cycloplegic
3. Administer an antibiotic
4. Patch the eye

2. CHEMICAL AND PHYSICAL INJURIES

A. Chemical Injuries

Chemical burns are quite common. They can be caused by either acid or alkali and usually occur in a laboratory or industrial plant. Regardless of the type of causative agent, chemical burns need immediate attention. An acid immediately precipitates the superficial tissue proteins and generally does not penetrate deeply into the eye. The damage is limited to the superficial layers of the cornea or conjunctiva and is immediate. There are no later effects such as cell disruption or tissue softening. On the other hand, alkali burns are much more serious. Alkali penetrates the cornea, the anterior chamber, and even the retina within a very short period of time. Penetrating alkali disrupts living cells and softens the tissue. Laboratory experiments show that an alkali-burned cornea contains broken-down collagen. The extent of injury of a chemical burn is related to the nature and concentration of the chemical agent. In general, the higher the alkali pH, the more serious is the injury.

SIGNS AND SYMPTOMS: In general, not only the conjunctiva and the cornea, but the eyelids and the surrounding skin also are involved in a chemical injury. The skin and the lids can be whitish (pale) and appear necrotic. Coagulation of the corneal tissue causes opacity of the cornea and, therefore, appears to be whitish and opaque (Fig. 5-2). The conjunctiva, if severely injured, is pale because it is ischemic. Pain can be severe, or none at all, depending on the damage of the sensory elements of the cornea. In most cases, the vision is severely impaired.

TREATMENT: Irrigation of the eyes and the surrounding tissue is the immediate treatment for chemical burns. As more time elapses between injury and decontamination, the prognosis worsens. One should not wait for a sterile, physiologic mild acid or alkali solution, but should wash out the chemical agent with tap water immediately. The fornices of the conjunctivas must be swept with wet cotton applicators; the eyelids should be everted and washed. Solid

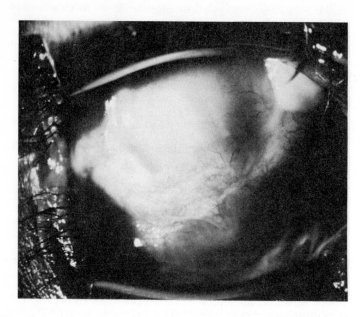

Fig. 5-2. An eye two months after alkali burn. The cornea is white and vascularized.

particles or crystals should be removed either by a cotton applicator or by a pair of forceps. Most ophthalmologists do not recommend irrigation for a long period of time if acid is the chemical agent causing the injury.

In the case of an alkali burn, the initial lavage should be followed by continuous irrigation with physiologic solution. At least 1000-2000 ml of normal saline 0. 9% should be used for at least one hour. Conservative approach recommends continuous irrigation for 24 hours. It was recently demonstrated that irrigation for long periods of time does not eliminate any more chemical agents from the ocular tissues. The best advice is to examine the pH in the conjunctival sac; if it is alkaline, continue the irrigation until the pH is restored to normal, or at least close to normal (tears have a pH of between 7. 3 and 7. 7).

After lavage, cycloplegics, mydriatics, and antibiotics are administered into the conjunctival sac. Atropine 1% or hyoscine 0. 3%, and neosynephrine 10% eyedrops are used to dilate the pupil and to prevent massive adhesions between the lens and the iris (posterior synechiae); also, they reduce the symptoms of secondary iridocyclitis. Chloromycetin, bacitracin, or Garamycin eye ointment is applied to prevent infection. Discomfort may be reduced with occasional administration of topical anesthetics. Frequent use of topical anesthetics is not recommended since they inhibit healing. If the pain is severe, systemic analgesics should be administered, the injured eye should be patched, and the patient must be hospitalized. The use of topical corticosteroids in chemical injuries is controversial.

COMPLICATIONS AND PROGNOSIS: Chemical burn caused by acid has a relatively good prognosis. The cornea and conjunctiva may be damaged seriously but the posterior segment of the eye rarely suffers from the injury. The ultimate prognosis of vision is relatively good.

Alkali burns are serious. Extensive destruction of conjunctiva and cornea is not unusual. In an alkali-burned cornea, collagenase is produced by cells which repopulate the damaged cornea (that is, epithelium). Collagenase attacks unprotected collagen of the cornea which causes ulceration, or even perforation, of the cornea. For this reason, collagenase inhibitors are used in the alkali-burned cornea starting one week after injury. Cysteine or acetylcysteine is used by many ophthalmologists. Cysteine is administered as a 0.2 molar solution, a few drops every four hours.

The outer layers of the ocular tissue as well as the inner aspect may suffer severely from the chemical agent; alkali may penetrate into the retinal tissue and destroy all the sensory elements, thus causing complete blindness. In general, chemical burns are not treated surgically in the emergency room. Tissue destruction becomes evident only a few days later. Surgery is usually not indicated during the first few weeks following an alkali burn. The only surgery of an emergency nature is therapeutic corneal graft after corneal perforation. Replacement of conjunctiva by buccal mucosa or corneal graft for optical reasons can be performed only several months after injury. Complicated cataract or secondary glaucoma is a common complication after chemical injuries. Surgery of any kind for alkali burns has a very poor prognosis.

B. Physical Injuries

ULTRAVIOLET RADIATION

Ultraviolet radiation is the most common form of radiation injury. Natural sunshine, sunlamps, and welding arcs are the more common causes of this type of injury. Usually the corneal epithelium is injured. The prognosis of such an injury is good. Permanent impairment of vision from ultraviolet radiation is not common.

SIGNS AND SYMPTOMS: The patient presents himself with severe pain, photophobia, and blepharospasm usually several hours after exposure. The latent period between the time of injury and the appearance of the symptoms may be from six to ten hours. The conjunctiva is chemotic and diffuse punctate fluorescein staining of the

cornea is present. Visual acuity may be normal or slightly deteriorated. Diffuse corneal haze may be seen in a severe case of industrial injury. Spastic miosis may develop. The pain may be relieved
by the application of topical anesthetics for a short period of time.

TREATMENT: Short-acting cycloplegic drops such as tropicamid
1% (Mydriacyl) or cyclopentolate 0. 5% (Cyclogyl) should be administered to relieve pain due to secondary iritis. Topical antibiotic
drops or ointment such as chloromycetin, bacitracin, or neomycin
will prevent infection. The eye should be patched for one or two
days. Analgesics also should be used to relieve the pain.

INFRARED RADIATION

Prolonged exposure to infrared radiation occasionally may produce
superficial keratitis. The so-called glassblower cataract is caused
by multiple exposures of infrared radiation, but this is not considered an ocular emergency.

SIGNS, SYMPTOMS, AND TREATMENT: The signs, symptoms,
and treatment of infrared radiation are the same as those of ultraviolet radiation.

THERMAL BURNS

A contact burn is not a common injury in civilian life. Thermal
burns usually effect the eyelids. Marked edema and redness of the
lids are seen. Because of the lid reflex closure, the cornea is
rarely affected. Accidents arise from flying objects such as the
lighted end of a cigarette. If the lid burn is so severe that lid closure is impaired, the exposed cornea must be covered with antibiotic ointment until a plastic surgery procedure can be performed to
replace the destroyed tissue. A corneal burn should be treated with
topical antibiotics and short-acting cycloplegics.

IONIZING RADIATION

Exposure of tissue to ionizing radiation is always followed by a latent period before any sign of reaction occur. The latent period
varies and depends on the dose of radiation. Occasionally, clinical
symptoms occur several weeks after injury; thus, ionizing radiation
is not always an emergency.

The conjunctiva and the cornea are considered to be more radiosen-
sitive than other tissues. The lens, uvea, retina, and optic nerve
also may suffer from ionizing injury.

SIGNS AND SYMPTOMS: The conjunctival reactions to radiation are
hyperemia, circumcorneal injection, and watery discharge. Mucopurulent discharge is not an uncommon complication. Visual acuity
may be normal or deteriorated.

The earliest clinical sign of radiational damage of the cornea is hy-
poasthesia. Radiation keratitis results in the loss of epithelium

resembling superficial punctate keratitis or superficial ulcers. Occasionally, interstitial keratitis and aseptic corneal necrosis may develop.

Clinical lesions of the uvea include vascular dilatation and tissue edema.

Hemorrhages in the retina, papilledema, and thrombosis of the central retinal vein are very rare complications of radiation injury.

Radiational cataract is always a late complication. The first clinical sign is the appearance of pepper-like opacities at the posterior pole of the lens in the plane of the capsule.

TREATMENT: The treatment of radiation injuries is symptomatic. A cycloplegic such as Cyclogyl 1% or homatropine 5% and an antibiotic such as chloromycetin 1%, gentamicin 1%, or tetracycline 1% should be administered to reduce signs of active iritis and to prevent infection.

3. CONTUSION AND CONCUSSION INJURY TO THE EYEBALL

Contusion and concussion injury can be classified as follows:

A. Contusion injury
B. Concussion injury due to tissue conduction
C. Concussion injury due to air conduction (Fig. 5-3)

A. Contusion injury of the eye is damage caused by direct contact with the eyeball by any one of a large variety of blunt objects, for example, a stone striking the eye directly, or a fist.

B. Concussion injury refers to a blow not directly striking the eye. An injury to the head is the most common cause of concussion injury of the eye by tissue conduction. The striking force hits the head and the waves of this force are conducted to the eye through tissue, namely the bone and the orbital fat.

C. Concussion injury conducted by air occurs in the case of an explosion. The waves come from an explosion far away from the eye. The waves hit the cornea and are transmitted to the other ocular tissues, causing many kinds of injury to the eyeball.

The results of contusion and concussion injuries are variable. They may cause damage to the anterior segment of the eye as well as the posterior segment. Very often the extent of damage shortly after injury is unknown. Careful follow-up is necessary in most cases to evaluate the final damage. Some signs such as hemorrhage or dislocated lens are evident immediately after injury; however, others, such as cataract, may develop later. The emergency room examination must first exclude the possibility of rupture of the eyeball. (Signs of perforating injury are described in the chapter entitled "Penetrating and Perforating Injuries".)

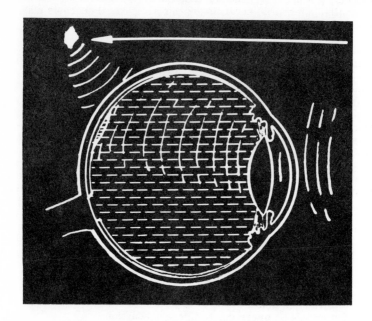

Fig. 5-3. Artist's drawing illustrating waves causing:
  a) concussion injury by air conduction, and
  b) concussion injury by tissue conduction.
  The waves are transmitted to the posterior pole and
  cause edema of the macula.

Concussion injury also can be classified according to the damage
caused to the ocular tissue. Concussion injury can cause:

  1. Molecular disturbances
  2. Vascular reactions
  3. Gross tissue changes

1. Molecular disturbance refers to disruption of the physiologic activity of cells due to trauma. Macroscopically, nothing can be
   seen. Microscopic examination sometimes reveals pathologic
   changes such as cromatolysis of certain cells. If this type of injury occurs in the macular area of the retina it may cause reduced visual acuity.

2. Vascular reactions are the more visible and more serious effects of a concussion injury. The trauma causes primarily vaso-
   paralysis; the blood flow in the affected area slows down. As a
   consequence of this, the endothelial cells are damaged and fluid
   escapes from the blood vessels, causing tissue edema. Edema
   of the retina is a good example of this type of injury.

3. Gross tissue changes are the most serious effects of the concussion injury. The striking force ruptures and disintegrates ocular
tissues. Mechanical tearing of vessel walls and other similar
changes occur. These changes are apparent mainly in the retina
and the choroid and cause serious intraocular hemorrhages. This
chapter will discuss only those pathologic conditions in which the
globe remains intact; however, some of these pathologic findings
may be present in a perforating injury as well. If the striking
force is mild, the globe remains intact. Occasionally, the contusion injury is so severe as to cause rupture of the eyeball.

Contusion or concussion injury may cause:
    A. Ecchymosis, subconjunctival hemorrhage
    B. Corneal lesions (opacities and rupture of membranes)
    C. Hyphema
    D. Iridodialysis, traumatic aniridia, changes in accommodation
       and refraction, and changes in the pupil
    E. Ciliary body detachment and traumatic iridocyclitis
    F. Recession of the anterior chamber angle, and other conditions
       causing concussion glaucoma
    G. Subluxation or dislocation of the lens and cataract
    H. Herniation of the vitreous into the anterior chamber
    I. Vitreous hemorrhage
    J. Rupture of the choroid, hemorrhage of the choroid, and trau-
       matic choroiditis
    K. Retinal hemorrhage and edema
    L. Retinal detachment
    M. Rupture of the eyeball
These injuries may appear separately or in combination.

A. Ecchymosis, Subconjunctival Hemorrhage: Ecchymosis is a
contusion injury of the eyelids. Hemorrhage and edema are present
in the eyelids. No special treatment is required is these are the
only conditions present. The hemorrhage and edema will disappear
gradually within a few weeks.

Hemorrhage from conjunctival and episcleral vessels may occur
without any or with only minimal laceration of the conjunctival tissue. Sometimes a large amount of blood coagulates under the conjunctiva causing a black ring around the cornea. Surgical evacuation
of such a clot is very often unsuccessful. The hemorrhage will dissolve within two weeks. No special treatment is required for this
condition. The use of antibiotic drops or ointment is advisable to
prevent possible secondary infection.

B. Contusion and Concussion Injury of the Cornea: Concussion injuries of the cornea may be of two types: 1) concussion necrosis,
2) laceration of tissue.

Direct impact by a blunt object may cause edematous opacities of
the corneal epithelium or endothelium. Concussion may cause edematous changes in the substantia propria forming a typically disc-
shaped or ring-shaped opacity of 2-3 mm in size. Occasionally,

folds of Bowman's or Descemet's membrane, or both, can be observed after a concussion or contusion injury.

A more diffuse and massive edema of the cornea may be seen if the injury causes tears in Descemet's membrane. Very often there is a break in the endothelium layer if the tear occurs in Descemet's membrane. This condition may result in permanent cicatricial opacities. Complete rupture of the entire cornea is extremely rare.

SIGNS AND SYMPTOMS: Pain, photophobia, lacrimation, blepharospasm, and reduced visual acuity might be present in case of a corneal injury due to concussion or contusion.

TREATMENT: No specific treatment for a concussion or contusion injury of the cornea is available. The routine emergency treatment includes a mild cycloplegic such as Cyclogyl 0.5%, an antibiotic such as chloromycetin 1%, and patching the eye.

C. Hyphema: Blood in the anterior chamber is called hyphema. The blood may fill the whole anterior chamber or only part of it. If the patient rests in a sitting position, the blood settles in the inferior portion of the anterior chamber. It is important to remember that a patient with hyphema is very often somnolent. Lack of alertness is particularly true in children. The exact mechanism of this somnolence or lethargy is unknown. However, brain concussion or other head injury must be considered also in such a patient, especially when trauma occurs to both the eye and the head.

TREATMENT: The patient must be hospitalized -- bed rest is necessary. The head should be elevated at least 60° and, if the patient is restless, sedation is indicated. In case of pain, analgesics should be used. Both eyes should be covered to provide maximal rest to the eyes. Local administration of a cycloplegic such as atropine 1% or homatropine 5% provides additional rest to the iris and ciliary body and reduces the effect of secondary iridocyclitis. Not all ophthalmologists agree on this point; some do not instill any medication in the eye in a case of hyphema. Also, the use of pilocarpine 2% eyedrops has been recommended as treatment for hyphema.

An elevated intraocular pressure indicates the presence of secondary glaucoma. It should be treated with a carbonic anhydrase inhibitor such as Diamox and with a hyperosmotic agent such as glycerol or mannitol. The method of administration and the amount of medication to be used is discussed in the chapter on glaucoma.

LATE COMPLICATIONS AND THEIR TREATMENT: Secondary hemorrhage from broken vessels may occur from the third to fifth day following injury. This type of hemorrhage is sometimes more serious than the primary hemorrhage. Secondary glaucoma with severe pain is not an unusual complication.

An eye with hyphema should be examined daily. Long-lasting hyphema may cause blood staining of the cornea. Blood pigment enters the cornea causing a brown discoloration of Descemet's membrane. Corneal staining is most likely to appear if both elevated intraocular pressure and extensive hyphema are present.

Surgical intervention, which means the evacuation of the blood from the anterior chamber, is indicated when either of two conditions obtains: 1) the conservative treatment of secondary glaucoma has proved ineffective, and 2) staining of the cornea is evident.

D. Iridodialysis; Traumatic Aniridia; Changes in Accommodation and Refraction; Changes in the Pupil: Iridodialysis (Fig. 5-4) is the disinsertion of the iris from the ciliary body and may occur in association with hyphema or with other pathologic conditions due to blunt trauma. After the initial period of rest no treatment is usually required. Occasionally, the iridodialysis is so extensive that the iris drops down, occluding the visual axis and interfering with useful vision. Diplopia and visual confusion may be present. In these cases, surgical intervention (that is, suturing the iris) is indicated several weeks or months after injury, when the eye is quiet and its condition is stabilized. If the root of the iris is completely torn from its attachment to the ciliary body, the condition is called traumatic aniridia. A complete hyphema usually accompanies this traumatic lesion. After absorption of the blood, a shrunken grey body can be seen in the anterior chamber. Also, complete retroflexion or inversion of the iris may occur in a severe concussion injury. No treatment is indicated in such cases. No medication is effective to correct the deformity.

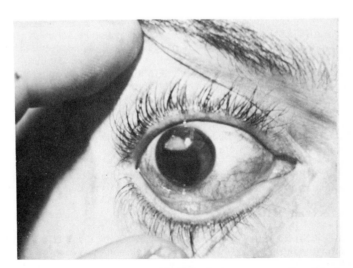

Fig. 5-4. Eye after trauma. Iridodialysis is seen nasally. The lens is cataractous and dislocated.

After blunt trauma, paralysis of the pupil may occur. The pupil may be dilated and may react to light. The accommodation can be impaired as well. This condition, called traumatic mydriasis may persist for several days and, occasionally, for weeks. A spastic miosis is an immediate constant sequel to a blunt trauma. The constriction of the pupil is intensive in nature and is usually transient. The exact mechanism of traumatic miosis is not completely understood. In some cases it can be explained to be due to sympathetic paralysis resulting from an injury to the skull or neck region.

Sometimes the pupil is irregular after trauma, due to rupture of the sphincter muscle of the iris. Irregularity of the pupil may be temporary or it may be permanent, lasting for the patient's lifetime.

Trauma to the eye is usually followed by inflammation of the uveal tissue. Traumatic anterior uveitis also causes constriction of the pupil.

After a blunt trauma, changes in the refraction may occur. Transient, or sometimes permanent, hypermetropia is not uncommon. It is believed that traumatic hypermetropia is due to injury to the ciliary nerves or the ciliary muscle itself.

Traumatic myopia also is a common consequence of trauma. It is mainly transient (from -1.0 diopter to -6.0 diopters). In most cases of traumatic myopia the ciliary spasm is responsible for the myopia.

E. Ciliary Body Detachment, Traumatic Iridocyclitis.
Ciliary Body Detachment: Dysfunction of the ciliary body following concussion injury is not an uncommon complication.

SIGNS AND SYMPTOMS: Low intraocular pressure and reduced visual acuity are the early signs of ciliary body detachment. The anterior chamber appears to be shallow. On fundus examination, prominence of the peripheral fundus is seen. The optic disc is usually edematous and macular edema also may be present.

Hypotony may result from a) damage to the ciliary body epithelium, and b) ciliary body detachment (traumatic cyclodialysis). Usually, hypotony due to ciliary body detachment lasts longer than that due to ciliary body epithelium damage.

TREATMENT: Hospitalization and bed rest are necessary. Topical administration of a cycloplegic such as Cyclogyl, 1%, three times a day, and a steroid such as prednisone, 30-60 mg a day by mouth, are recommended.

PROGNOSIS: Ciliary body detachment following trauma is usually temporary; however, it may last for weeks or even months. The end result might vary from complete recovery to severe glaucoma or complete loss of function of the affected eye.

Traumatic Uveitis

Traumatic uveitis is a very common condition. It may occur in any contusion injury or after severe corneal injury including foreign body, laceration, or chemical injury, and is more severe in a heavily pigmented eye. Traumatic uveitis is not present immediately after injury, but appears a few hours or days after the injury.

SIGNS AND SYMPTOMS: The patient's visual acuity is reduced. Photophobia is common and often severe. The patient suffers from pain of the affected eye, headache also may occur, the conjunctiva is red, the episcleral vessels are engorged, and the pupil is constricted.

TREATMENT: The primary cause of the traumatic uveitis must be treated, if necessary (removal of the foreign body or rust ring). A short-acting cycloplegic such as cyclandelate 0.5% (Cyclogyl), and a mydriatic (Neosynephrine 10%) should be administered. If the uveitis is severe, the drops should be used 3-4 times a day. Dark glasses or patching of the affected eye help to relieve the discomfort. Topical steroid drops also should be considered in the event that the corneal epithelium is intact and there is no sign of bacterial or fungal infection.

F. Recession of the Anterior Chamber Angle and Other Conditions Causing Glaucoma: The effect of a concussion or a contusion injury on the intraocular pressure may be dramatic and sometimes a determining factor concerning the fate of the eye. The rise in tension usually develops immediately or shortly after the injury. In 20% of cases it may develop more than one week later. The cause of concussion glaucoma is not well understood. It may be complex and not necessarily an injury to one particular part of the eye.

Recently, recession of the anterior chamber has been mentioned as a common cause of post-traumatic elevated intraocular pressure. Biomicroscopic examination of these cases shows areas with a wide, open angle of the anterior chamber. It is believed to be due to displacement of certain structures such as the ciliary muscles, from the trabecular meshwork area. In addition to these macroscopic changes, the normal histology of the trabecular meshwork and the whole drainage system are injured as well.

Thrombosis of ciliary veins and endothelial changes in the vortex veins are also among the possibilities which can cause elevated intraocular pressure after contusion or concussion injury. Subluxation or dislocation of the lens, herniation of the vitreous, and intraocular hemorrhages are responsible in different ways for elevated intraocular pressure after trauma. These conditions are discussed elsewhere in this chapter.

TREATMENT: Initial treatment of concussion glaucoma is not different from other types of secondary glaucoma. To reduce intraocular pressure, carbonic anhydrase inhibitors and hyperosmotic agents can be used immediately after diagnosis. Diamox 250 mg, four times a day by mouth, or glycerol 1 gm per kg body weight, two or three times a day, might be effective to reduce intraocular pressure. In addition to the above, miotic eyedrops such as pilocarpine 2% should be administered 3-4 times a day. Occasionally, sympathomimetic eyedrops such as epinephrine or norepinephrine 1% (Eppy 1%), administered twice a day helps to reduce the intraocular pressure.

G & H. Traumatic Cataract; Traumatic Dislocation of the Lens; Herniation of the Vitreous into the Anterior Chamber: Cataract development after contusion of the eyeball is not unusual and may occur without any detectable damage to the capsule. The exact mechanism of this type of cataract is not known. Generally, the cataract must be extracted several months after injury.

Blunt trauma to the eyeball can cause subluxation or complete luxation of the lens (see Fig. 5-4). The striking force tears the zonules holding the lens in place behind the iris in the center of the pupil. If the lens drops into the vitreous body, the condition is called complete dislocation of the lens. If part of the zonules remain intact, the lens is pulled slightly toward the intact zonules. This condition is called subluxation of the lens.

The anterior chamber may deepen in these conditions and iridodonesis (trembling of the iris) also can be seen. The hyaloid face of the vitreous may be disturbed and the vitreous may herniate into the anterior chamber (Fig. 5-5). Occasionally, the lens may become partly or completely dislocated into the anterior chamber. This situation may cause a shallow anterior chamber. Also, the lens may touch the posterior surface of the cornea. Very often, secondary glaucoma accompanies these conditions. The most common mechanism of secondary glaucoma is pupillary block. The aqueous cannot pass from the posterior chamber through the pupil into the anterior chamber because the lens, or the vitreous, occludes the pupil completely or partially.

TREATMENT: When dislocation of the lens or herniation of the vitreous causes an elevated intraocular pressure, immediate surgical intervention is not indicated. The patient should be hospitalized and the secondary glaucoma should be treated. The condition of the eye should be completely evaluated, including visual acuity, intraocular pressure, and other pathologic conditions caused by the trauma. In general, complete dislocation of the lens into the vitreous cavity rarely requires lens extraction. If the lens is partly dislocated and occludes the pupil, causing secondary glaucoma, surgery is indicated. Herniation of the vitreous through the pupil causes elevated intraocular pressure and also calls for surgery. Lens extraction combined with anterior vitrectomy is the correct type of treatment.

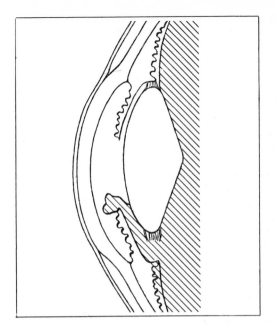

Fig. 5-5. Artist's drawing showing rupture of zonules, rupture of the hyaloid face, and herniation of vitreous into the ante- rior chamber.

I. Vitreous Hemorrhage: Vitreous hemorrhage caused by trauma is a serious condition. The hemorrhage may originate from retinal vessels or from the uvea. The route of absorption, damage to dif- ferent ocular tissues, and the early and late complications after vitreous hemorrhage are discussed in more detail in the chapter on "Sudden Loss of Vision" under the section entitled "Vitreous Hemor- rhage."

SIGNS AND SYMPTOMS: If no other pathologic condition accompa- nies vitreous hemorrhage there is little, if any, pathology present in the anterior segment of the eye. The pupil may be more dilated in the affected eye than in the fellow eye. The patient's visual acuity is markedly decreased, sometimes reduced to light perception only. On fundus examination, no details of the fundus can be seen because of vitreous haze. Occasionally, the vitreous hemorrhage is so se- vere that the red reflex of the fundus cannot be elicited. On exami- nation, the reflex is black.

TREATMENT: There is no specific treatment for vitreous hemor- rhage. Rest in a sitting position may be helpful because the blood corpuscles will gravitate to the lower part of the vitreous and, in this way, the central portion of the vitreous body will clear up sooner. Bilateral patching is useful; however, if the patient is rest- less with both eyes occluded, it is considered best to abandon the bilateral patching. The effectiveness of an oral or a subconjunctival enzymatic agent such as Varidase (streptokynase and streptodornase enzymes), fibrinolysin, or Chymolase (pancreatic enzyme) is questionable.

Mechanical removal of opaque vitreous, that is, partial or total vitrectomy, is advocated by many ophthalmic surgeons. This may be considered only if the absorption of blood has been insufficient for a period of a few months. This type of surgery is not an easy procedure and has many hazards.

PROGNOSIS: The patient may resume his usual activities a few weeks after injury but vigorous motion of the head and eyes must be avoided. Absorption of blood from the vitreous body may take many weeks or months. Occasionally, the blood may organize in the vitreous causing retinal detachment and serious loss of visual acuity.

J. Rupture of the Choroid: Severe contusion or concussion injury of the eyeball can cause rupture of the choroid. At the time of injury only vitreous or retinal hemorrhage can be seen, with marked deterioration of vision. After absorption of the hemorrhage a whitish, semicircular scar with mild pigmentation can be seen at the posterior pole (Fig. 5-6). In more than four-fifths of the cases, the fissures are on the temporal side of the disc. A nasal crescent is rare and horizontal ruptures are seen only occasionally. If the whitish scar transects the papillomacular nerve bundles (the nerve fibers between the optic disc and the macular area), the resulting visual acuity is always poor (20/200-20/400). Occasionally, the scar is outside the macular area and causes only minor changes in visual acuity but does cause a visual field defect.

TREATMENT: The only treatment required is bed rest for a few days after injury.

Choroidal Hemorrhage

Hemorrhages of the choroid is a relatively common sequel to contusion injury and may occur without rupture of the Bruch's membrane or the layer of the pigment epithelium. The hemorrhage can spread between the choroid and the sclera, detaching the choroid from the sclera. On fundus examination, the area of choroidal hemorrhage seems to be elevated and has a dark brown color. The vision may or may not be affected, depending on the site and extent of the damage.

TREATMENT: No immediate effective treatment is known for choroidal hemorrhage. Bed rest, with the head elevated, for several days, is the conventional treatment.

Chorioretinal Rupture

Occasionally, a simultaneous rupture of both the choroid and the retina may occur. If the retina also is torn, the hemorrhage may extend into the vitreous. This type of injury is more common in war when the striking force is great. At the time of injury the fundus rarely can be seen. Later, proliferating chorioretinitis, originating from the site of injury, often causes retinal detachment by traction.

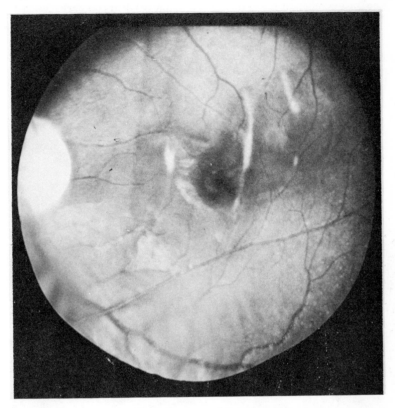

Fig. 5-6. Rupture of the choroid

Traumatic Choroiditis

Traumatic injuries may occur in blast injuries. It is believed that first the striking force causes tissue necrosis. The necrotic tissue initiates vascular reaction which causes hemorrhage. Considerable degrees of pigment proliferation and subsequent atrophy of the uveal tissue is the usual course.

The symptoms of traumatic choroiditis are the same as those of mechanical rupture of the choroid. The treatment is the same as in choroidal rupture, that is, bed rest for a few days.

K. Retinal Hemorrhage and Edema: Shortly after injury, hemorrhage or edema may be found in the retina. Hemorrhages can be subhyaloid, preretinal, in the superficial layers of the retina, or in the deeper layers of the retina. The more anterior the retinal hemorrhage, the brighter is the red color. Deep hemorrhages are rather greyish or bluish-red. The hemorrhages may occur in different shapes depending on the depth (Fig. 5-7). Round hemorrhages are located deep in the retina, while flame-shaped hemorrhages are more superficial.

Retinal edema is the extravasation of fluid from the blood vessels. It is believed that the primary blow causes a reflex vasospasm, that is, functional occlusion of the fine vascular network of the retina. As a result, there is anoxia and malfunction of the endothelial cells of the vessels. The anoxic endothelial cells are not able to retain the fluid inside the vessels and so the fluid escapes into the surrounding tissue.

Edema of the retina may appear at the site of the injury or, more commonly, at the posterior pole. This condition is called also Berlin's edema, or commotio retinae.

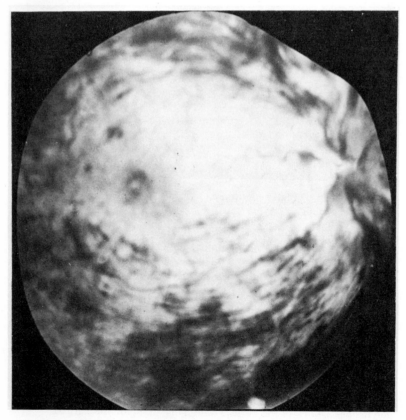

Fig. 5-7. Retinal hemorrhages after contusion injury of the eyeball

Despite the retinal hemorrhages, the visual acuity can remain very good unless the hemorrhage occurs in the macular area. Edema of the retina, especially edema at the posterior pole, causes reduced visual acuity. The prognosis of retinal hemorrhage and edema is unpredictable. In certain cases the edema or the hemorrhage, or both, absorb quickly with no significant damage to the vision. In other cases the edema disappears only weeks after the injury; in these cases, the visual acuity will be markedly reduced.

TREATMENT: No specific treatment is known for retinal hemorrhage or retinal edema. Several ophthalmologists insist on bed rest for several days; however, there is no proof that bed rest improves these conditions. If the retinal edema persists for longer periods of time with no sign of improvement, oral steroid treatment might be beneficial. Many ophthalmologists treat retinal edema with high doses of steroid (prednisone 120 mg per day) immediately after the injury.

L. Traumatic Retinal Detachment: Retinal detachment due to trauma occurs in most cases after the injury. There are two main groups of detachments to be considered concerning trauma. In one group, a retinal hole or disinsertion occurs at the time of injury. These holes, or disinsertions, are responsible for retinal detachment at a later stage.

In the other group, there are no holes in the retina at the time of injury. Vitreous hemorrhage occurs and, later, the vitreous hemorrhage leads to traction band formation in the vitreous body. These traction bands pull on the retina, either tearing it or detaching it. Other conditions which may cause retinal detachment are retinal edema and hemorrhage. The retina becomes necrotic and cystic in those areas with the edema or hemorrhage and finally retinal holes develop. These holes occasionally may cause retinal detachment at a later stage (Fig. 5-8).

In most cases of contusion or concussion of the eye the prominent ophthalmoscopic appearance of the fundus is the presence of multiple hemorrhages and extensive retinal edema. Retinal tears can be seen only occasionally. Most of the holes or tears are peripheral to the equator and are not visible with a direct ophthalmoscope. It is difficult to differentiate between areas of severe retinal edema and retinal detachment occurring immediately or shortly after the initial trauma.

TREATMENT: Traumatic retinal detachment should be treated differently from other types of detachment. No immediate surgery is required. Bed rest for one week with bilateral patching is the most advisable immediate treatment. Most surgeons prefer to postpone surgery until the hemorrhages and edema have subsided. Therefore, practically speaking, traumatic retinal detachment is not an ophthalmologic emergency. Careful re-examination and re-evaluation after concussion and contusion injury, with or without retinal detachment, should be an almost routine requirement. The emergency room physician should instruct the patient to undergo such an examination.

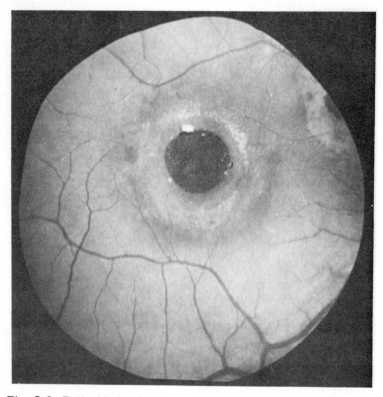

Fig. 5-8. Retinal hole of traumatic origin at the macula. The retina is detached around the hole.

M. Rupture of the Eyeball: Rupture of the eyeball due to blunt trauma occurs quite often. The signs, symptoms, and management of the ruptured globe will be discussed in the chapter entitled "Penetrating and Perforating Injuries of the Eyeball."

RETINOPATHY DUE TO DISTANCE INJURY
(PURTSCHER'S DISEASE)

A patient involved in a car accident or suffering from head or chest injury may present with a special type of retinopathy which is called "Purtscher's disease" or "angiopathia retinae traumatica." The eyes are not involved directly in the accident and, except for the retina, do not show much pathology. The pathogenesis of the disease is not known. Purtscher explains the changes in the retina to be caused by "pronounced rise in the pressure of the cerebrospinal fluid, which is transmitted to the perivascular lymph space of the central vessels in the optic nerve. This pressure mechanism causes the escape of blood corpuscles and plasma into the retinal tissue."

SIGNS AND SYMPTOMS: The condition appears within the first two days after injury. The visual acuity may or may not be impaired, depending on the degree of involvement of the macular area. The eye shows minimal pathologic damage except in the retina. On fundus examination, superficial round, white, patchy exudates are seen close to the retinal veins. Small linear hemorrhages can be seen all around the posterior pole. Edema of the perimacular area is common. In general, the arteries are narrow and the veins are congested.

TREATMENT: The treatment is expectant.

PROGNOSIS: The fundus changes gradually disappear within a few days or weeks. The vision may or may not return to normal, depending on how severely the macular area was involved.

LATE COMPLICATIONS AFTER BLUNT TRAUMA TO THE EYEBALL

PHACOLYTIC GLAUCOMA

A lens which has been traumatized can develop a cataract. Occasionally, the cataract may be hypermature. The cortical material of the lens becomes liquified and leaks through the lens capsule into the anterior chamber. This lens material flares up a characteristic macrophage reaction in the anterior segment of the eye. Proteinaceous material and cellular debris clog the outflow channels of the aqueous humor. This condition, the combination of severe anterior uveitis and extremely high intraocular tension, is called phacolytic glaucoma.

Phacolytic glaucoma may occur also without any history of trauma; however, it is more common in a traumatized eye.

SIGNS AND SYMPTOMS: The patient suffers from headaches, the eye is extremely painful, the vision might be light perception only, the intraocular pressure is high, the conjunctival and subconjunctival vessels are engorged, and the cornea is hazy. If the anterior chamber can be seen through the cornea, severe flare and a large number of cells can be observed and a cataractous lens is seen behind the constricted pupil.

TREATMENT: Phacolytic glaucoma is one of the rare conditions when emergency cataract extraction is indicated. Conservative treatment does not improve the condition of the eye and the high intraocular pressure may cause permanent blindness within a short period of time. The intraocular pressure must be reduced by a hyperosmotic agent such as intravenous urea or mannitol, and then the cataractous lens should be removed.

PROGNOSIS: The postoperative course is benign in most cases. The inflammation subsides quickly and the intraocular pressure returns to normal. Visual acuity may vary between useful vision and light perception, depending on how long the intraocular pressure was elevated and how much of the optic nerve was damaged.

CHAPTER 6

TRAUMA: PART II

PENETRATING AND PERFORATING INJURIES OF THE EYEBALL

A penetrating or perforating wound of the eye is relatively common. The wound may be a small puncture or an extensively large wound. A child may be injured in the playground or in school; an adult engaged in industry or in household duties may have an accident which can cause perforation of the eyeball. A great number of eye injuries in civilian life occur at the time of an automobile accident. War injuries are the largest contributors to perforating ocular injuries.

The causative agents are innumerable; knives, needles, pens, pencils, pins, and sharp toys are among the more common ones in children. Flying bodies, small particles, glass fragments, and sharp instruments and tools account for eye injuries among adults. These injuries require immediate and careful attention; surgery is essential when a penetrating or perforating injury of the eyeball is suspected.

The following procedure is indicated, regardless of whether or not the wound is large or small or the clinical picture is complicated by prolapse of intraocular content :

1. History
2. Eye examination
3. X-ray examination
4. Tetanus prophylaxis and antibiotic therapy
5. Surgical intervention (if necessary)

1. History of the injury requires an exact description of the accident or injury; this may help considerably in evaluating the extent and seriousness of the injury.

2. Examination of the eyeball requires careful examination. No pressure should be applied to the globe when a penetrating or perforating injury is suspected. Minimal eye examination should include vision, estimation or measurement of intraocular pressure, examination of the anterior segment, and at least an attempt to examine the posterior segment. If the examination is painful, or if it might endanger the integrity of the globe (as in the case of a large wound), the extent of the injury should be evaluated completely under local or general anesthesia. Under no circumstances should visual acuity examination be neglected, especially for medico-legal reasons.

3. X-ray examination of the injured eye is necessary to determine the presence and location of a radiopaque intraocular foreign body. This examination is described in detail in the chapter on emergency ophthalmologic radiology.

4. Tetanus prophylaxis must be performed as soon as possible.
Cases of tetanus caused by eye injuries have been described in the
past. Also, prophylactic antibiotic therapy is absolutely essential.
Ocular infection after injury is very common and the early start of
antibiotic therapy is very effective.

5. Surgical intervention: Successful surgical intervention and the
possibility of preserving the useful function of the eye are possible
only if the above-mentioned four points are completed. Improper
preparation for surgery, if it is necessary, may bring fruitless results with regard to visual acuity, and perhaps even survival of the
eye. As an example, immediate closure of the visible wound may
cause serious complications if an intraocular foreign body was not
detected previously and was not removed from the globe.

The terminology and classification of penetrating and perforating
eye injuries is very confusing. The following classification is widely
used and well accepted.

(1) Penetrating injury refers to partial tissue damage of the outer
coat of the eye (cornea or sclera). An example of this injury is when
a foreign body with low velocity enters into the sclera and remains
impacted among the lamellae, or a sharp object cuts through two-
thirds of the cornea leaving Descemet's membrane intact. This type
of injury is not a true through-and-through wound of the sclera or
cornea.

(2) Perforating injury refers to complete discontinuation of tissue
through the entire thickness of the coat of the eyeball; in other
words, an open wound is present through the cornea or the sclera.
Perforating injury can be divided into three groups:

1. Perforating injury without retained intraocular foreign body
2. Perforating injury with retained intraocular foreign body
3. Double perforation of the globe (Fig. 6-1)

The term "laceration" also is used commonly, especially when a
through-and-through corneal (or scleral) wound is present.

SIGNS OF PERFORATION OF THE EYEBALL: The following signs
may be indicative of perforation of the globe:

1. Reduced visual acuity
2. Reduced intraocular pressure (hypotony)
3. Change in depth of the anterior chamber
4. Displacement of the pupil or change in the shape of the pupil
5. Visible wound of the cornea or the sclera
6. Prolapse of ocular tissue (uvea, lens, vitreous, retina)
7. Chemosis of the conjunctiva

In the case of a perforation, not all of the above-mentioned signs
are always present. On the other hand, these signs are not pathog-
nomonic for perforating injury, but may occur in other conditions.

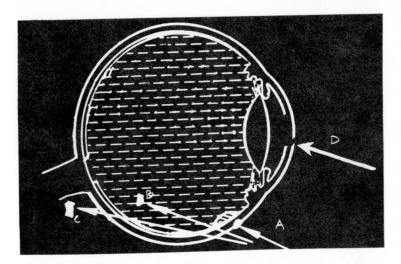

Fig. 6-1. Artist's drawing, a) penetrating injury to the eyeball. A foreign body is impacted among the scleral lamellae; b) perforating injury with retained intraocular foreign body; c) double perforation with a foreign particle; d) corneal perforation.

For example, low intraocular pressure may present after blunt trauma to the eye with no perforation. Also, chemosis of the conjunctiva may occur in many conditions with no perforation of the globe.

The depth of the anterior chamber changes in almost all cases of perforated injury. It becomes shallow if the perforation is in the anterior segment, since the aqueous humor escapes through the perforation. The anterior chamber becomes deep if the perforation is posterior and ocular tissue protrudes through the wound.

The pupil can change its shape and position if anterior uveal tissue (iris, ciliary body) extrudes through the wound, whether or not the wound is visible.

IMMEDIATE MANAGEMENT OF PENETRATING OR PERFORATING INJURY: Life-saving measures have priority over eye care; however, immediate minimal care of a penetrating or perforating injury of the eye may not interfere with life-saving measures and, therefore, should not be neglected or unduly postponed.

The injured eye should be treated in the emergency room after thorough and careful examination, as already described in this chapter. The treatment can be divided into two parts:

1. General and supportive therapy
2. Ocular treatment

The general and supportive therapy should include massive antibiotic treatment, tetanus prophylaxis, analgesics, sedation, and antiemetic, if necessary.

All medications should be administered intramuscularly or intravenously. Oral intake of food or beverages should be discontinued immediately. These measures will permit the patient to be anesthetized safely for surgical repair when optimal conditions for surgery are present.

Nausea or vomiting should be suppressed by proper medication, as vomiting increases the intraocular pressure which may result in unnecessary prolapse of intraocular tissue through the open wound; also, it might cause hemorrhage from the damaged tissue.

The psychologic effect of an eye injury also should be considered; the patient should be adequately sedated until the damaged globe can be repaired.

Topical treatment of the injured eye in the emergency room should be minimal. Instillation of antibiotic eyedrops such as Chloroptic (chloromycetin 0.5%), Garamycin, or Neosporin, and patching of the eye are essential. However, mydriatic or miotic eyedrops should not be used prior to surgery as the effect of these medications might make the necessary surgical repair more difficult.

The use of any kind of ointment is not recommended when an open wound is present, as it might penetrate the open globe.

As movements of both eyes are associated, and movements of the uninjured eye may cause undesirable movement of the injured globe, bilateral patching should be considered if the psychologic condition of the patient permits.

SURGICAL REPAIR OF THE RUPTURED GLOBE: The different types of penetrating and perforating injury of the anterior segment and their surgical management are outlined and discussed in Chapter 7. This chapter describes only the surgical management of a globe ruptured behind the ora serrata. This type of injury and its management differ somewhat from a wound in the anterior segment because of the presence of the retina posterior to the ora serrata. Of course, each traumatic injury is different and, therefore, only a brief general description of the surgical repairs are described.

A peritomy of the conjunctiva is performed. The area of the suspected scleral rupture is completely exposed and Tenon's capsule and other episcleral tissue is excised. After exposure of the scleral wound, uveal tissue, vitreous, or retina may be present at the site of the traumatic wound. Debridement of the sclera is rarely necessary, if at all. Other devitalized tissue must be excised and removed from the lips of the scleral wound. Vital uveal prolapsed tissue should be replaced in the globe by gentle pressure with a blunt spatula. The edges of the scleral wound must be matched very carefully. Incarceration of uveal tissue between the lips of the scleral wound is undesirable and considered a faulty surgical repair. Interrupted sutures are suitable more often than continuous sutures for repair of a traumatic wound. The suture material used varies according to the training and experience of the ophthalmic surgeon. Fine mersilene, silk, or monofilament nylon sutures are all equally suitable for repair of the sclera.

After proper closure of the scleral wound, surface diathermy or cryocoagulation is applied around the injured area. This seems to be helpful in preventing retinal detachment in the future. If the sclera is badly lacerated, or a considerable amount of tissue is missing, cadaver sclera or fascia lata might be sutured on and around the damaged area to reinforce the sclera and to prevent post-traumatic scleral staphyloma.

If a considerable amount of vitreous is lost after surgical repair of the traumatic rupture, the intraocular pressure must be restored by injecting air or saline into the vitreous cavity. A silicone explant or cadaver sclera sutured to the globe at the site of the injury indents the sclera and minimizes vitreous traction on the retina (see Fig. 6-9).

Antibiotics should be administered immediately after surgery. Subconjunctival injection of Garamycin 40 mg (gentamicin), or another broad-spectrum antibiotic is necessary. A systemic broad-spectrum antibiotic must be continued for at least 7-10 days to prevent endophthalmitis. It is the author's opinion that the use of corticosteroids is advisable to reduce postoperative and post-traumatic reactions.

INTRAOCULAR FOREIGN BODIES

The retention of a foreign body within the eye is not a very common injury. However, an intraocular foreign body should be suspected if periorbital or ocular tissue damage or wounds are visible. The emergency room physician must rule out the presence of an intraocular foreign body in each case, regardless of the patient's history concerning the injury.

Intraocular foreign bodies can be divided into two main groups:

    A. Metallic foreign bodies
    B. Nonmetallic foreign bodies

Metallic foreign bodies can be further subdivided into two groups:

    1. Magnetic foreign bodies
    2. Nonmagnetic foreign bodies

Both metallic and nonmetallic foreign bodies include inert substances which cause very little, if any, reaction within the eye. Such inert substances include gold, silver, platinum, or tantalum. Nonmetallic inert substances are stone, glass, porcelain, carbon, and certain plastics.

An irritative material can be either metallic or nonmetallic. Metallic materials are lead, zinc, nickel, aluminum, copper, and iron. There are many irritative nonmetallic substances, including vegetables, cloth particles, cilia, and eyelid particles.

The eye reacts to a retained foreign body in various ways, depending on the composition of the particle. Some are inert for an indefinite period of time, while others may enter into chemical combination with the tissue and cause severe reaction. The same type of foreign body may react differently in different ocular tissues. In general, a foreign body in the anterior chamber or in the lens causes much less reaction than does one in the posterior segment. The ocular reaction may be of three types:

A. Certain nonorganized material causes no specific reaction. Its presence in the tissue causes mechanical irritation which, in turn, encapsulates the foreign body. The reaction is only exudative and fibroplastic in type.

B. Other nonorganized material may interact with the tissue of the eye in chemical reaction which finally produces specific or nonspecific damage.

C. Organized material sets up a proliferative reaction with formation of granulation tissue and giant cells.

The injury caused by a foreign body is determined also by the momentum with which it enters the eye. A large foreign body travelling with sufficient velocity disrupts the whole globe. A small particle with sufficient velocity enters the globe but the main structure of the globe is preserved.

In civilian life, the velocity of the striking foreign body is usually low; however, in war injury or in blast injury, the velocity of the foreign particle is high. The site where a foreign body comes to rest within the eye varies with its point of entry and its velocity. Therefore, intraocular foreign bodies in the anterior segment are more common in civilian life, such as industrial and car accidents; in the posterior segment,. in war casualties.

The size of the retained foreign body varies. The smallest foreign body that may enter the eye is at least 0. 25 mm x 1. 0 mm x 1. 0 mm in size (Fig. 6-2). The largest intraocular foreign body may measure 3. 0 mm x 3. 0 mm x 3. 0 mm, and weigh 500 mg. When a larger-sized foreign body enters the eye, the eye is hopelessly disorganized as is the case in a war injury when a bullet destroys the entire globe.

From the clinical point of view, the most important characteristic of a foreign body is its magnetic properties. If a foreign body has a high content of iron, it is magnetic and its removal is relatively easier than that of a nonmagnetic foreign body. The incidence of intraocular magnetic foreign body in industrial accidents is relatively

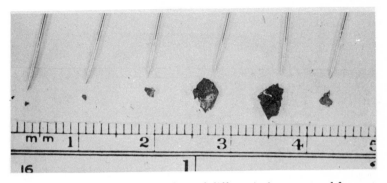

Fig. 6-2. Metallic foreign bodies of different size removed from patient's eyes

high and, therefore, the percentage of successful removal of intraocular foreign bodies is also high.

Various techniques are available to determine the presence, consistency, and location of an intraocular foreign body. They are as follows:

1. Ophthalmoscopy
2. Slit lamp
3. X-ray
4. Magnet
5. Metal detector
6. Ultrasound

Direct visualization by slit lamp and ophthalmoscopy (particularly indirect ophthalmoscopy) are the means best suited to detect the presence of an intraocular foreign body (Fig. 6-3). Unfortunately, however, the media of the injured eye is rarely clear enough to allow careful examination and to determine the presence or absence of a foreign body. Perforation of the lens capsule can lead to rapid cataract development, thus making impossible proper examination of the posterior segment.

Direct visualization of the anterior chamber with the slit lamp and the gonioprism is sometimes useful to discover an intraocular foreign body in the anterior chamber or in the chamber angle. A transparent foreign body such as glass may be discovered only after careful slit-lamp examination.

In addition to the previously mentioned examination methods, radiologic techniques should be used in all cases of suspected intraocular foreign body regardless of whether or not a foreign body is detectable with direct observation. In the case of a perforating injury, multiple foreign bodies often may be retained. Occasionally, not

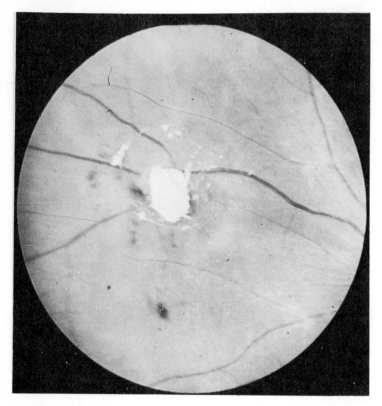

Fig. 6-3. Intraocular foreign body adherent to the retina

all intraocular particles can be seen by direct visualization, and an x-ray examination will detect most of them.

The exact procedure as to how to perform a radiologic examination and to determine whether the foreign body is intraocular or extra-ocular, is described in the chapter on ophthalmologic radiology.

Radiology may be helpful also in determining the nature of the foreign body. For example, different metals show different shadows on x-ray films. Iron shows a stronger shadow than does aluminum; therefore, by performing an x-ray examination of the globe, one may learn about the chemical constitution of the foreign body. Only an experienced radiologist can make such a determination.

In the case of a traumatic eye injury, the use of a magnet to locate a foreign body containing iron also is helpful. The magnet (Fig. 6-4)

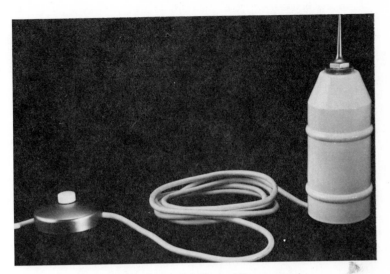

Fig. 6-4. Powerful Storz Atlas magnet

can be employed as a diagnostic instrument to determine the presence of a foreign body within the eye. When a powerful magnet is brought into close contact with the globe containing a magnetic particle, the latter is drawn towards the pole of the magnet. If the particle is drawn toward a sensitive area such as the ciliary body, the resulting pain betrays its presence subjectively. This method of diagnosis, however, is not recommended routinely since a small movement of the particle inside the eye may cause serious and unnecessary additional injuries.

In the absence of other diagnostic means, namely, x-ray, the magnet can be used when verification of the diagnosis is urgently needed.

If the magnetic foreign body entered the eye many weeks prior to examination and has become encapsulated, no movement may occur and no pain may be elicited. A negative result is, therefore, not always conclusive, while a positive result may cause additional injury.

The principle of the metal detector method depends on the fact that if there is an alternating current through a primary circuit, a current is induced in secondary coils by induction. If the voltages in the secondary coils are equalized, no current flows between them, but if in this state the instrument approaches a metallic body, the balanced inductance is disturbed and a difference in potential is created in the secondary circuit. This difference results in a flow of current which may be recorded by variations in the tone of a loudspeaker or by the deflection of the needle of a voltmeter.

The amount of current varies with the magnetizability of the particle, its size, and its distance from the metal detector. A magnetic metal effects profoundly the magnetic field created around the instrument, but a nonmagnetic metallic substance also can be detected.

The Berman locator (Fig. 6-5) is one of the more popular instruments of this type used in ophthalmology and is very sensitive. It has a detecting range for iron of 10 times the diameter of the particle, that is, a 1-mm diameter of iron is detectable at 10 mm. In the case of a nonmagnetic metal, the sensitivity is only one to two times the diameter of the particle, that is, a 2-mm diameter of aluminum can be detected at 2 mm distance while a 2-mm diameter of copper can be detected at a distance of 4 mm, copper being a more dense metal. (The thickness of the sclera is approximately 1 mm!)

Ultrasonography is one of the newer types of instrumentation used to search for foreign bodies. This method is still in the development phase. It may help considerably in the diagnosis and prognosis of eye injuries with or without retained intraocular foreign body. Recently, the usefulness of an ultrasonic transducer for localization and ultrasonically directed forceps for removal of nonmagnetic in-

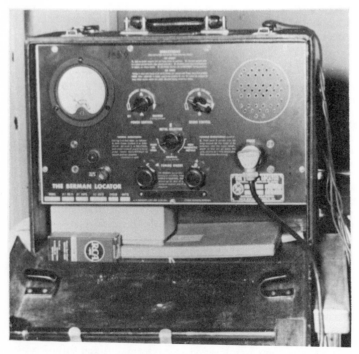

Fig. 6-5. Berman metal detector

traocular foreign bodies was reported. Trained skilled personnel is necessary to operate these instruments and to interpret the results. Because it is not available in many institutions and its use is not as yet routine, this book will not discuss the use of ultrasound in any detail.

GUIDELINES FOR TREATMENT: Once the presence and the location of an intraocular foreign body are established, the decision to treat the case surgically or conservatively must be made. In most cases of intraocular foreign body, the prognosis is guarded. Two important goals of the treatment must always be considered:

1. Preservation of the eyeball
2. Restoration of useful vision

Enucleation or evisceration immediately after injury is rarely necessary. In most cases, recovery and restoration of vision is unpredictable at the time of injury. The persistence of light perception is a strong indication to make every effort to remove the foreign body and to preserve the globe. If there is very little hope of preserving the globe because of severe injury caused by the foreign body, an attempt to remove the foreign body and to repair the globe is still indicated. This approach does not jeopardize the patient's well-being or the vision of the other eye. If enucleation should prove to be necessary, it can be done several days later. Additional contraindication to immediate enucleation or evisceration is the psychologic trauma. Enucleation or evisceration following injury causes additional unnecessary psychologic trauma to the already emotionally disturbed patient.

It is absolutely necessary that the eye and the entire orbit on the injured side be handled carefully prior to surgical intervention. Occasionally, the eyeball must be closed temporarily before performing the procedures necessary to locate the intraocular foreign body. This is necessary in order to prevent the prolapse of intraocular tissue during radiologic or ultrasonic examination of the globe.

Injured intraocular tissue, in particular, uveal tissue, tends to bleed. Therefore, during diagnostic procedures such as physical examination or x-ray examination, the tissue must be handled gently to prevent secondary bleeding.

As mentioned previously, the reaction of the eye to a foreign body depends largely on the chemical nature of the foreign body and its position within the eye. The physician must be aware of the risk involved in leaving a relatively inert foreign body in the eye and to compare this risk to the surgical risk involved in its removal; finally, he must decide what type of treatment, surgical or conservative, promises better visual acuity. In general, it is hazardous to leave in the eye a foreign body which contains iron or copper. Within a few days copper can cause severe intraocular inflammation which may destroy the eye. A retained foreign body of iron or of copper may cause also late occurring syndromes such as sidero-sis or chalcosis, respectively. Therefore, early removal of a for-eign body of iron or copper is strongly recommended.

On the other hand, a small piece of stone lying on the lower portion of the retina may cause very little disturbance to the vision and very little inflammatory reaction in the eye. In the long range, the stone will be encapsulated by fibrous tissue with very little possibility of late complications or inflammation. Therefore, considering the surgical trauma involved in removing the stone and the complica-tions occurring from an inert intraocular foreign body, it is almost always advisable to leave the intraocular particle untouched.

To summarize, the risks involved in leaving a foreign body in the eye must be weighed against the danger of removing it surgically.

The location of the foreign particle in the eye is also of considerable importance in the final decision as to how to treat the injured eye. For example, a foreign object visible in the anterior segment usu-ally is not difficult to remove. The surgical trauma is minimal and, therefore, the decision between surgery and conservative treatment is easily reached. On the other hand, it is more difficult to reach a decision when the same particle is in the vitreous.

The decision to remove the foreign body should be made before the particle becomes encapsulated by fibrous tissue. The encapsulation of the foreign body takes a few days rather than a few hours. This gives the physician enough time to perform the necessary diagnostic tests. Therefore, there is no necessity for the immediate removal of the particle; the decision and the treatment should be carefully planned and executed within a few days after the occurrence of the injury.

METHODS OF REMOVAL OF AN INTRAOCULAR FOREIGN BODY

Basically, there are two routes for foreign body removal:

1. Anterior route
2. Posterior route

In the anterior route, the foreign body is removed through a cor-neal opening or a corneoscleral incision anterior to the iris and the lens. This route is suggested in cases where the foreign body is visible and direct manipulation will cause little damage to the tissue. If the foreign body is in the anterior segment and visible, it can be successfully extracted with the use of forceps. The anterior route can be utilized also to remove a magnetic foreign body located in the posterior segment (Fig. 6-6).

This method of extraction utilizes a magnet to draw the foreign body into the anterior chamber. When the foreign body is visible, it is removed from the anterior chamber by means of forceps or a magnet. With this technique, it is not necessary to locate the foreign

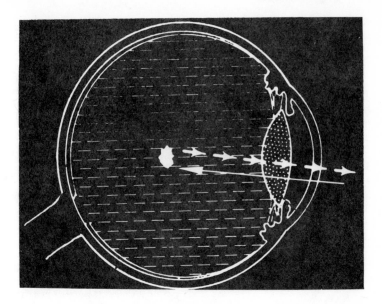

Fig. 6-6. Anterior route of foreign body removal. Straight line
shows the route of entry of the foreign body. Dotted line
shows the route of extraction.

body precisely. Maximal dilation of the pupil is required. The anterior route of extraction is indicated only in the presence of a large corneal wound and a traumatic cataract.

The anterior route is less advisable in cases where the foreign particle is in the posterior segment and not visible. There is great risk of damaging the uveal tissue and the lens when the magnet is used to pull the particle against living tissue.

If the lens is intact, it is almost always contraindicated to use the anterior route of extraction when the foreign particle is located behind the lens because of the potential damage to the lens capsule and the zonules.

The posterior route is the extraction of the foreign particle located behind the lens and iris diaphragm. This route can be subdivided also into two groups:

    A. Extraction at the pars plana area
    B. Extraction at the site of the foreign body

A. Most surgeons choose to remove a magnetic foreign body through the pars plana. This site is convenient also to introduce an instrument into the globe to remove a nonmagnetic foreign body from the vitreous cavity (Fig. 6-7). Here, the retina is thin and firmly attached to the underlying tissue. There is little risk of

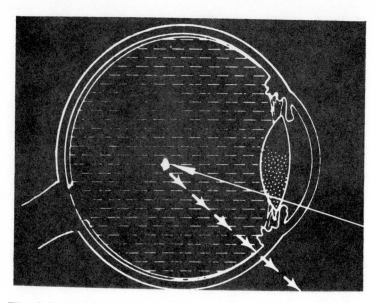

Fig. 6-7. Foreign body removal through the posterior route, pars
plana area. Straight line shows the route of entry. Dotted
line shows the route of extraction.

retinal detachment due to the surgical manipulation. Also, the
area is relatively avascular; there are no choriocapillaries in
this area and, therefore, hemorrhage resulting from the surgical intervention rarely occurs.

B. If the foreign body is deeply embedded in the retina (also in certain cases of nonmagnetic foreign body), the particle cannot be
extracted through the pars plana area. Therefore, the incision
should be made at the site of the foreign body, thus providing the
most convenient access to the embedded particle. Extraction of
a foreign body through the sclera at the posterior pole has the
potential risk of hemorrhage and retinal detachment, regardless
of the preventive measures the surgeon is obliged to take. Surgery at the posterior pole can result in irreparable damage to
vital structures, namely, the retina and the vitreous.

In conclusion, there is considerable controversy regarding the extraction of a foreign body by either the anterior or the posterior
route. Each has its advantages and its contraindications. Thus,
each case involving an intraocular foreign body should be dealt with
individually.

SURGERY - THE ANTERIOR ROUTE: In any surgery of this type,
general anesthesia should be used. Local anesthesia is not desirable
and should be used only if general anesthesia is contraindicated or
not available. If the foreign body is metallic, an attempt should be
made to remove it with a magnet.

The tip of the magnet is brought close to the corneal wound. The current is turned on. The magnet draws the foreign body into the anterior chamber where it can be removed by forceps. Alternatively, one can continue to pull the foreign body with the magnet until the foreign particle attaches to the tip of the magnet. The rest of the operation is the same as described in detail in the chapter on anterior segment reconstruction surgery.

THE POSTERIOR ROUTE:

a) Pars plana approach: The pars plana area corresponding to the foreign body is exposed. If the foreign body is magnetic, it is pulled toward the pars plana by the magnet taking the shortest route through the eye. Once the foreign body is at the inner surface of the globe, it should be located by means of a Berman locator. A deep scleral incision or a deep scleral window penetrating to the outer surface of the choroid is made. This incision or window should be large enough to accommodate the foreign body. One or two 6-0 or 7-0 silk or mersilene sutures are passed through the lips of the surgical wound. These sutures are used also to expose the surgical area. Surface diathermy is applied to the area surrounding the window to wall off the area of surgery and to the exposed uveal tissue. The tip of the magnet is placed against the exposed uvea, and the current is turned on. The magnet draws the foreign body which cuts its own way out of the eye. The surgeon punctures the uvea with a small nonmagnetic instrument or needle. This reduces the actual force of the magnet needed to extract the foreign particle. After the extraction, the incision is closed by the preplaced traction sutures. Additional sutures may be used to close the incision properly. The scleral incision should be cleaned of vitreous debris before its final closure.

In the case of a nonmagnetic foreign body in the middle of the vitreous cavity, the surgeon may choose to enter the globe at the pars plana. The scleral incision is made large enough to introduce the extracting instrument into the eye. The incision should be deep and should extend to the outer surface of the uveal tissue. Two 6-0 silk or mersilene sutures are passed through the lips of the incision to expose the area. Surface diathermy is applied to the surrounding area and to the exposed uveal tissue. The uvea is opened and the forceps (or other instrument) is inserted in the globe. Simultaneous indirect ophthalmoscopy aids to locate the foreign particle. After the extraction, the preplaced sutures are tied. The vitreous debris is removed from the incision and additional sutures are used for sufficient closure of the incision.

b) Extraction at the site of the foreign body: After the administration of anesthesia, an area of sclera corresponding to the foreign body is exposed. The foreign body is located by means of a Berman locator (this is necessary only if the foreign body is metallic). If the media are clear, indirect ophthalmoscopy is used for precise location. A deep scleral window penetrating to the outer surface of the choroid is prepared (Fig. 6-8). Preplaced 6-0 or 7-0 silk sutures are passed through the lips of the incision. Surface diathermy is applied to the surrounding area and to the exposed uveal tissue. This

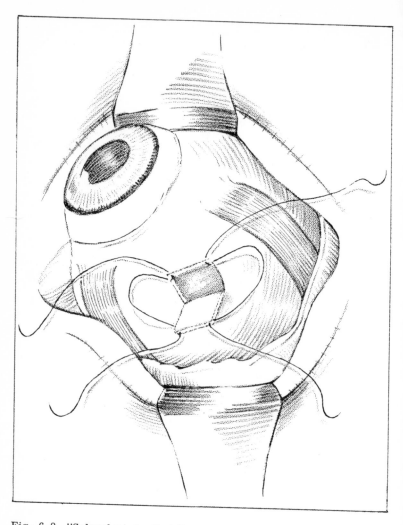

Fig. 6-8. "Scleral window" at the site of the intraocular foreign body.

will reduce the possibility of bleeding from the choroid and walls off the area of surgery. In the case of a metallic foreign body, an attempt should be made to remove the foreign body by magnet by placing the tip of the magnet on the exposed uvea and activating the magnet by turning on the current. If the foreign body is magnetic, it will be drawn out of the globe through the uvea. The surgeon may puncture the uvea with a nonmagnetic instrument to help the foreign body make its way out of the globe.

If the foreign particle does not respond to the magnetic force, the uveal tissue is opened at the site of the retained object. The foreign body is then removed by applying light pressure around the area. If the foreign body is not removed, an instrument may be inserted through the incision. The movement of the instrument in the globe should be controlled by direct visualization. It is not advisable to enter the globe with an instrument if one cannot control the movements visually since vital tissues can be damaged irreparably. Following extraction, the vitreous is removed from the wound and the wound is then closed using 6-0 silk or mersilene interrupted sutures. A silicone explant or cadaver sclera is sutured to the globe at the site of surgery to minimize postoperative vitreous traction on the retina (Fig. 6-9).

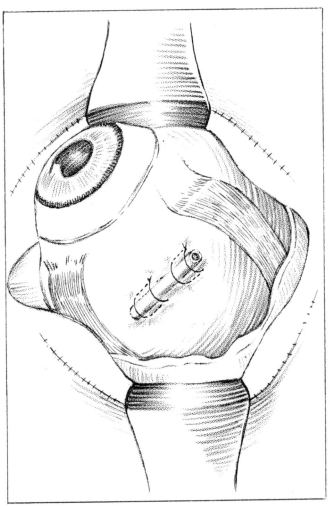

Fig. 6-9. Cadaver sclera sutured on the globe at the site of surgery.

In all cases of intraocular foreign body, antibiotics should be administered. Subconjunctival injection of 200 mg Ampicillin, 0.5 gm Staphcillin (methicillin), or 40 mg of Garamycin is given at the end of the surgical procedure. In addition, broad-spectrum antibiotics are administered topically and systemically for at least seven days. The use of corticosteroids is extremely helpful to reduce postoperative reaction of the vitreous body. Oral administration of prednisone 30-60 mg daily is necessary for 2-3 weeks postoperatively to prevent vitreous traction caused by inflammatory reaction.

LATE COMPLICATIONS OF PERFORATING INJURIES AND PROGNOSIS OF INTRAOCULAR FOREIGN BODIES

The literature reports only a small number of cases wherein a foreign body was successfully removed and the visual acuity is followed for many years. The end results of cases where the foreign body has been allowed to remain in the globe are extremely difficult to assess in terms of vision. The presence of a chemically active body is almost always disastrous. The presence in the eye of a foreign particle which contains iron or copper is particularly hazardous.

Siderosis is a late complication of an intraocular foreign body containing iron. This is a delayed chemical reaction of the ocular tissues to the metallic particle. It is a chronic degenerative process resulting in blindness. The seriousness of the disease depends on the ferrous content of the foreign particle. The less the ferrous content, the less the tendency to siderosis. The exact chemistry of siderosis is not yet understood. It is believed that iron molecules enter the cells. Once within the cells, the iron combines with protein to form an insoluble protein-iron complex which is responsible for the death of the affected cells. It has been observed that certain cells have a special affinity to absorb more iron molecules than others. The most dense deposit of the metal occurs on the anterior surface and the musculature of the iris, the trabecular meshwork of the anterior chamber, the subcapsular epithelium of the lens, the epithelium of the ciliary body, and the peripheral retina.

Siderosis occurs from two months to two years after injury. Diminution of vision, increased dark adaptation time, night blindness, and concentric contraction of the visual field are definite signs of the disease. Electroretinography (ERG) may help considerably in the early diagnosis of the disease and the prognosis of an eye containing an iron particle. Karpe divided the ERG changes into three stages. In Stage 1, both the "a" waves and "b" waves are increased. If the foreign body is removed at this stage, the electric response of the affected eye is normalized. In Stage 2, the "a" wave is still increased but the "b" waves are diminished. In Stage 3, both "a" and "b" waves are extinguished. At this stage, all the above-mentioned definite clinical signs of siderosis are present. It is believed that removal of the foreign particle in a late stage rarely helps to stop progression of siderosis.

In later stages of the disease, the deterioration of visual acuity and other signs of the disease are graver and, finally, complete amaurosis develops.

Chalcosis, a disease similar to siderosis, is induced by copper molecules. The preferential deposit of copper is either in or on the limiting membranes of the eye rather than intracellular, as in the case of siderosis. The clinical appearance of the disease is less dramatic and the prognosis is not nearly as poor.

Sometimes an eye can retain a copper-containing foreign body for long periods of time without significant loss of vision.

The clinical appearance of chalcosis is characterized by 1) a greenish-blue ring in the peripheral cornea located in Descemet's membrane, 2) a sunflower cataract in the anterior capsule of the lens, 3) impregnation of the zonular fibers, 4) metallic particles in the aqueous humor, 5) greenish coloration of the iris, 6) copper particles deposited in the vitreous and on the surface of the retina. A similar clinical picture can be observed in Wilson's disease (hepatolenticular degeneration) which is actually an endogenous chalcosis.

Specific treatment for chalcosis is still not available and ultimate visual loss is likely from a retained foreign body containing copper.

SYMPATHETIC OPHTHALMITIS

Sympathetic ophthalmitis is a rare disease which may occur after a perforating injury of the eye, particularly if the uveal tissue is injured or prolapses and remains so for some time. The disease is a bilateral, granulomatous uveitis originating in the injured eye. The onset of inflammation in the fellow (uninjured) eye is usually within three weeks to two months after injury; however, inflammation in the fellow eye occurring from nine days to many years after ocular trauma have been reported. In untreated cases of iris or ciliary body prolapse, sympathetic ophthalmitis may occur in as high as 5% of cases. The incidence of this disease in modern ophthalmology, however, has diminished greatly. Prompt and precise post-traumatic surgery, early enucleation, if necessary, and the introduction of corticosteroid therapy account for the marked decline in the incidence of sympathetic ophthalmitis.

Corticosteroids given topically, subconjunctivally, and systemically after injury may prevent the development of the disease. Once the noninjured eye shows signs of granulomatous uveitis, it is doubtful whether enucleation of the injured eye is beneficial to prevent further progression of the disease. Untreated cases tend to be progressive and about 50% lose useful vision.

Previously it was stated that if a perforating injury is complicated by the retention of a foreign body, prophylactic enucleation is indicated. This was practiced especially if the foreign body was lodged in the ciliary body. However, observations after the Second World

War indicated that the incidence of sympathetic ophthalmitis following retention of a foreign body was relatively low. It is believed that
with the introduction of corticosteroids in modern ophthalmology the
relatively low incidence of sympathetic ophthalmitis is further reduced in cases of retained intraocular foreign bodies.

PHACOANAPHYLAXIS

Only rarely does an eye, subsequent to injury, develop a delayed
inflammatory reaction with granulomatous uveitis. The pathogenesis
of granulomatous uveitis is most likely the injury to the lens capsule at the time of injury and the escape of lens material, which
causes a phacoanaphylactic reaction in the eye. Phacoanaphylaxis is
probably similar in pathogenesis to that of sympathetic ophthalmitis. Granulomatous uveitis also may develop in the injured eye because of sensitivity to lens protein.

Systemic and local corticosteroids have been beneficial in a delayed
post-traumatic complication. Recently, the incidence of phacoanaphylaxis has been markedly reduced. Although the disease is not
entirely prevented, the final visual results are remarkably improved.

TRAUMATIC CYST

The development of cysts within the eye after a perforating injury
is not a rare complication. An organized foreign body retained within the eye may result in cyst formation. An epithelial implantation
cyst may follow a perforating injury. In the cornea, epithelial cells
grow into the wound or small fragments of the epithelium are detached and transplanted to another layer. Epithelial proliferation
may form a cyst in the anterior chamber. Sometimes several cysts
may coexist at the same time. Implantation cysts within the globe
are relatively rare and may be of two types, 1) pearl cysts, 2) serous cysts. The pearl cyst is a solid greyish-white body which becomes evident a few months or a few years after injury. The serous
cyst is more common. Its walls are more translucent and contain
yellowish fluid. Serous cysts may develop earlier than pearl cysts.
The diagnosis of these intraocular cysts is not always easy. Cysts
may cause iridocyclitis which may further complicate the clinical
picture. Secondary glaucoma may develop in an eye with an implantation cyst. The differential diagnosis between an intraocular cyst
and neoplasm may be extremely difficult. The history of perforating
injury is always an important factor in making the correct diagnosis. The treatment of these intraocular cysts is usually surgical.
Occasional reports appear in the literature regarding radiation
therapy for traumatic cysts. While the surgical removal of cysts is
sometimes successful, ultimate consequences of cysts are usually
serious.

BIBLIOGRAPHY

1. Braun, S. I. : Alkali burns of the cornea. Arch Ophthal 82:91, 1969.

2. Braun, S. I. : Prevention of the ulcer of the alkali burned cornea. Arch Ophthal 82:95, 1969.

3. Bronson, H. R. II: Non-magnetic foreign body localization and extraction. Amer J Ophthal 58:133, 1964.

4. Byron, H. M. : Ocular trauma. Eye, Ear, Nose, Throat Monthly 42:48, 1963.

5. Duke-Elder, S. : System of Ophthalmology, vol. XIV. Injuries. Henry Kimpton, London, and Mosby, St. Louis, 1972.

6. Easom, H. A. and Zimmerman, L. E. : Sympathetic ophthalmia and bilateral phacoanaphylaxis: A clinico-pathologic correlation of the sympathogenic and sympathizing eyes. Arch Ophthal 72: 9, 1964.

7. Gombos, G. M. : Ocular war injuries in Jerusalem during the 1967 Arab-Israeli conflict. Amer J Ophthal 68:474, 1969.

8. Gregorson, E. : Traumatic hyphema: Report of 200 consecutive cases. Acta Ophthal 40:192, 1962.

9. Guy, L. P. : Use of Berman locator in removal of magnetic intraocular foreign bodies. Arch Ophthal 36:540, 1946.

10. Hogan, M. J. and Zimmerman, L. E. : Ophthalmic Pathology: An Atlas and Textbook, 2nd ed. W. B. Saunders Co. , Philadelphia and London, 1962.

11. Hoefle, F. B. : Initial treatment of eye injuries. Arch Ophthal 79:33, 1968.

12. Karpe, G. : Early diagnosis of siderosis retinae by the use of electroretinography. Docum Ophthal 2:277, 1948.

13. Karpe, G. : Indications for clinical electroretinography. Arch Ophthal 60:889, 1958.

14. Marr, W. G. and Marr, E. G. : Some observations on Purtscher's disease; Traumatic retinal angiopathy. Amer J Ophthal 54:693, 1962.

15. McDonald, P. R. : Penetrating wounds of the eye. Trans Amer Acad Ophthal 60:812, 1956.

16. Moncreiff, W. F. and Schreribel, K. J. : Penetrating injuries of the eye. Amer J Ophthal 28:1212, 1945.

17. Newell, F. W. , Copper, J. A. D. , and Farmer, C. J. : Effect of BAL on intraocular copper. Amer J Ophthal 32:161, 1949.

18. Oksala, A. : Treatment of traumatic hyphema. Brit J Ophthal 51:315, 1967.

19. Paton, D. and Goldberg, M. F. : Management of Ocular Injuries. Saunders, Philadelphia, 1976.

20. Penner, R. and Passmore, J. W. : Magnetic VS nonmagnetic intraocular foreign bodies. Arch Ophthal 76:676, 1966.

21. Purtscher, O. : Angiopathia retinae traumatica, Lymphorrhagien des Augengrundes. Albrect V. Graefes Arch Ophthal 82: 347, 1912.

22. Runyan, T. E. : Concussive and Penetrating Injuries of the Globe and Optic Nerve. Mosby, St. Louis, 1975.

23. Schmöger, E. : Electroretinography in siderosis and chalcosis. Klin Mbl Augenheilk 128:158, 1956.

24. Snell, A. C. : Perforating ocular injuries. Amer J Ophthal 28: 263, 1945.

25. Stokes, W. H. : Unusual retinal vascular changes in traumatic injury of the chest. Albrect V. Graefes Arch Ophthal 7:101, 1932.

26. Symposium of the New Orleans Academy of Ophthalmology. Industrial and Traumatic Ophthalmology. Mosby, St. Louis, 1964.

27. Tower, P. : Traumatic choroiditis. Arch Ophthal 41:341, 1949.

28. Wilder, H. C. : Intraocular foreign bodies in soldiers. Amer J Ophthal 31:57, 1948.

29. Woods, A. C. : Clinical and experimental observation on the use of ACTH and cortisone in ocular inflammatory disease. Amer J Ophthal 33:1325, 1950.

CHAPTER 7

TRAUMA: PART III

NONPENETRATING AND PENETRATING INJURIES OF THE ANTERIOR SEGMENT

Types of Injuries and Surgical Management

INTRODUCTION

The immediate non surgical supportive therapy for lacerating trauma involving the anterior segment has been outlined in Chapter 6. The importance of the thorough examination of the globe in any lacerating injury, seemingly involving the lids alone, is again stressed. It is also reemphasized that repair of the anterior segment is not necessarily an emergency procedure. It may be delayed to permit repair of more generalized injury and also to permit the patient to be anesthetized safely for sufficient time to effect a good repair of the globe. Also, extensive orbital and lid lacerations accompanying an eye injury must be repaired simultaneously, since tissue swelling may make it impossible to approach the globe surgically for a considerable period. Therefore, it is important that the patient and the eye be in as satisfactory a state as possible before a surgical approach is made and this surgical approach should be an operating room, not an emergency room, procedure.

Particularly in the case of repair of lacerating injuries of the anterior segment, the use of an operating microscope and microsurgical instruments and suture materials is essential for the most effective repair. Since this equipment is not part of the usual emergency room surgical armamentarium, anterior segment surgery must be performed in the operating room. The surgical microscope and surgical instruments which are used to effect these repairs will not be outlined in this text since they are adequately described elsewhere. The author's preference is for a major zoom-type microscope and surgical instruments designed specifically for ophthalmic microsurgery. The suture material best suited to repair anterior segment lacerations, including those of the iris, is 22-micron or 13-micron monofilament nylon suture as currently manufactured by Ethicon under the trade name Ethilon. This is used on one of two needles, the longer 7.5 mm, GS-10, or the newer and shorter, 5.5 mm, GS-14 spatula needles. Unless otherwise specified, this suture material in one of the two sizes mentioned will be the only one recommended for use in the sections to follow.

TYPES OF INJURIES

Anterior segment injuries vary from simple nonpenetrating corneal lacerations to complete avulsion of and destruction of the anterior globe. We shall begin with a simple outline of the various types of injuries and then proceed with suggestions for their repair.

CORNEAL LACERATIONS

Simple corneal laceration (Fig. 7-1A) can be linear[2,3], irregular[1,4], or avulsing[5,6] with the lacerating implement entering either vertically or obliquely (Fig. 7-1B), in a particular injury. The incision may be partially penetrating or penetrating, or both. The anterior segment may be otherwise unharmed or the penetrating laceration may involve the iris. This latter can be either entirely internal (Fig. 7-2, A and B, left side) or prolapsed externally (Fig. 7-2, A and B, right side) with or without iris laceration. When incarcerated, iris sphincter or the dilator fibers, or both, can be included in the wound. It is evident that the more central the lesion, the less likely for peripheral iris to be prolapsed, and vice versa. Peripheral iris injuries are more liable to be lacerating because of the closer proximity of the iris to the cornea. In addition, they are more difficult to disengage from corneal laceration and more likely to form postoperative anterior synechiae even if apparently effectively released at surgery. If a simple incarceration of nonlacerated iris is seen immediately and there are no attendant generalized injuries preventing immediate repair, this can be considered an eye surgical emergency. The immediate repositioning of the iris with suturing of the corneal laceration can avoid iris necrosis. Delayed surgical repair makes reposition difficult or impossible as prolonged incarceration may produce sphincter or dilator paralysis and an irregular pupil.

Corneal laceration may be complicated also by an accompanying disruption of the lens (Fig. 7-3, A and B). If this occurs without iris involvement there is usually disruption of the anterior capsule only. A point-penetrating injury such as that caused by a wire may go through-and-through the lens (Fig. 7-3B), even to pierce the posterior globe, finally to enter the posterior orbit.

The lens may be dislocated without its being lacerated (Fig. 7-4B) or together with disruption of the anterior and, sometimes, the posterior capsule. Lens dislocation in the young patient is rare, but the older the patient, the weaker the zonular attachments to the lens, and lens dislocation may be seen more frequently. Vitreous then prolapses forward to become involved with the iris in the anterior laceration (Fig. 7-4, A and B). In the case of through-and-through penetration of the lens, with or without dislocation, vitreous is involved and may be seen often in the anterior segment or protruding through the wound with the lens material. In a laceration such as this, if the iris is involved, the traumatic penetration of the lens, when it is small, is sometimes obscured by the iris injury and may be missed by the surgeon even when operating under microscope magnification. The postoperative development of cataract, of course, indicates that lens trauma actually had occurred and was overlooked (Fig. 7-18). However, in a doubtful situation, the later management of a delayed developing traumatic cataract with an apparently intact capsule is preferable to immediate lens removal.

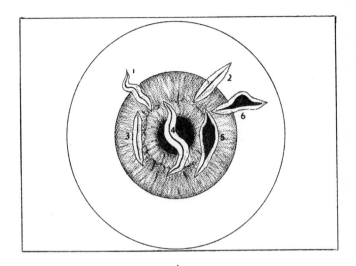

A

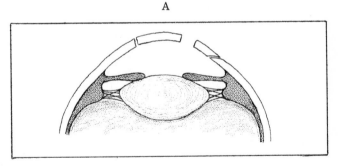

B

Fig. 7-1A. Diagrammatic representation of corneal and corneoscleral lacerations: (1) irregular corneoscleral laceration; (2) linear corneoscleral laceration; (3) linear
corneal laceration; (4) irregular corneal laceration;
(5) avulsing corneal laceration; (6) avulsing corneoscleral laceration.

Fig. 7-1B. Diagrammatic representation of vertical, oblique, and
avulsing corneal lacerations.

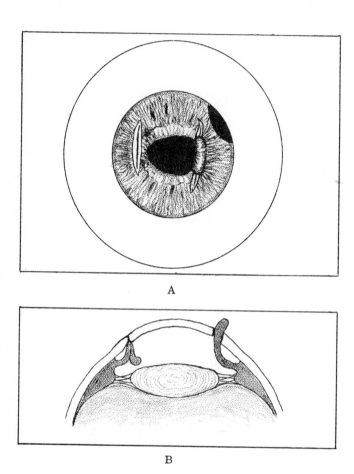

A

B

Fig. 7-2. A and B. Diagrammatic representation of a penetrating laceration with iris incarceration: (left) entirely internal; (right) iris prolapsed externally.

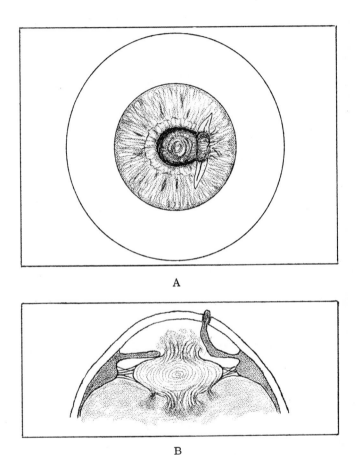

A

B

Fig. 7-3. A and B. Diagrammatic representation of corneal laceration with iris prolapse and disruption of the lens. (A) anterior view; (B) cross-section.

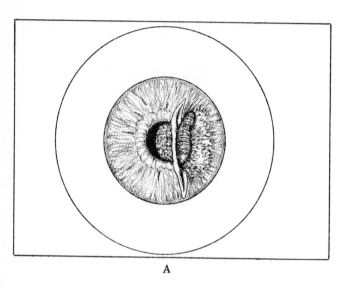

A

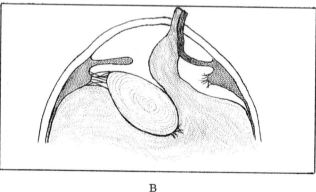

B

Fig. 7-4. A and B. Diagrammatic representation of corneal laceration with prolapse of iris and vitreous and dislocated lens. (A) anterior view; (B) cross-section.

The more peripheral the corneal lesion and iris trauma, the greater the likelihood that hemorrhage will accompany such compound injuries to the anterior segment. The extent of posterior injury can be completely obscured by blood and the laceration and its attendant posterior damage can be thoroughly evaluated and managed only at surgery.

SCLERAL LACERATIONS

Lacerations involving the anterior sclera can be simple or, as is the usual case, combined with corneal laceration (see Fig. 7-1A). They, too, may be linear [2], irregular [1], or avulsing [6] with through-and-through or partial penetration entering vertically or obliquely (see Fig. 7-1B). Because of its juxtaposition to the anterior scleral coat, the highly vascular ciliary body is almost invariably involved in anterior scleral lacerations and, as is the case with very peripheral penetrating injuries of the cornea, hemorrhage is the rule rather than the exception. Though laceration of the vitreous with presentation of vitreous through the wound is a common accompaniment of scleral injuries, traumatic damage to the lens is less frequent. Indeed, the globe may be partially, or even completely, collapsed as a result of vitreous loss through a scleral laceration and the lens can remain intact. Injuries posterior to the ciliary body and the pars plana will be considered elsewhere. These, however, may be merely extensions of anterior injuries. As a general rule, the more posterior the injury, the less the chance for survival of vision since complications involving the retina and vitreous tend to be more severe and less responsive to medical and surgical therapy.

MANAGEMENT - IMMEDIATE: Immediate management consists of medication for control of pain and the administration of a broad-spectral coverage of systemic antibiotics. In the emergency room, until adequate surgical therapy can be attempted, the patient should be sedated, his pain controlled, and have both eyes bandaged without pressure. The patient should be given nothing by mouth other than necessary medication in preparation for general anesthesia. When circumstances of the injury indicate the need, x-rays of the eye and orbit should be taken. If the presence of a foreign body is determined or suspected, a magnet or metal locator should be available at surgery to aid with its removal during the repair. A general evaluation of peripheral injuries by general medical and surgical personnel is essential to determine if the patient can be adequately and safely anesthetized for repair of his eye injuries. The importance of preserving the vision even in a badly injured patient cannot be overemphasized. Since the eyes represent more than half of the brain's function, the needless loss of an eye or eyes because of delayed or inadequate therapy can subsequently disable the patient more than many more immediately apparent peripheral injuries.

Without a doubt, one of the more important though controversial therapeutic agents used for treatment of lacerating injuries of the anterior segment is the corticosteroids. In the opinion of this author, administration of such agents may be delayed until the general condition of the patient and the condition of the injured eye can be evaluated, but no longer than 24 hours. Antibiotics must be given immediately, if no sensitivity is known or suspected or, at the least, simultaneously with the administration of corticosteroids in order to reduce the possibility of the steroid masking a serious uncontrolled infection. In many cases, the eye is lost because of too long a delay in the use of anti-inflammatory agents. It is essential that these agents be administered within 24 hours of the eye injury and continued after surgical therapy until the last vestiges of inflammatory reaction have disappeared from the repaired globe. Delay in administration of steroids is much more likely to result in loss of the globe than the rare sympathetic ophthalmia.

DELAYED MANAGEMENT: When the patient's general condition has been thoroughly evaluated and life-saving procedures effectively instituted, the general medical consultant should be asked to assure the ophthalmologist in writing that the patient is ready for anesthesia so that he may undertake surgical repair of the eye injuries. In any such potentially protracted and complicated microsurgical procedure, general anesthesia is preferable to local anesthesia if it can be administered safely to the patient.

It should be reemphasized that, in most instances, the definitive repair of a lacerating injury to the anterior segment is not an absolute emergency procedure. In an instance when severe general injuries threaten the patient's life, these must be dealt with first. When possible, repair of the eye injuries should be delayed to permit the use of general anesthesia so that a careful and complete primary repair can be performed. However, if at all possible, repair should be effected within the first 24 hours after the injury and no later than 48 hours after the injury. The deeper and more extensive the eye injury, the greater the post-traumatic inflammatory reaction and the greater the possibility of infection. Early debridement and repair will help to reduce the extensive inflammation and severe infection which can result from prolonged retention of damaged or necrotic tissue or infectious agents introduced at the time of injury. Since antibiotics and steroids take some hours to have their full effect, reparative surgery is best performed when antibiotic and antisuppressive therapy has reached its highest therapeutic level, 24-48 hours after injury. Microsurgical technique using fine instrumentation and nonreacting monofilament sutures should be used to minimize surgical trauma, as has been stressed earlier in this chapter, to reduce postoperative morbidity - the better to ensure late survival of the injured globe.

REPAIR OF CORNEAL LACERATION: When an adequate exposure has been obtained by speculum or lid sutures, the globe is immobilized with fixation sutures and a Flieringa ring. A careful inspection is made to determine the type and extent of the ocular injury. In the case of a simple corneal laceration, debridement is rarely necessary and even inadvisable, since small attached or even free pieces of lacerated cornea can be used as autografts to seal avulsing injuries. If they are removed and discarded in an overzealous debridement, it can become necessary to use homograft material which may not be readily available. Matching of the opposing wound edges should be done very carefully since linear displacement of the incision during suturing not only is surgically undesirable but can create unnecessary gross astigmatic errors in the healed cornea. Matching can be best accomplished by visually aligning slightly irregular portions of the laceration under high magnification, as in a jig-saw puzzle. When these areas appear to be in apposition, interrupted sutures are deeply placed, that is, to Descemet's membrane, to fix firmly the matched areas holding corneal laceration in position for linear closure (Fig. 7-5A). After the sutures are tied, the cornea is inspected carefully with the microscope and, if so equipped, with a keratometer to be certain that a large astigmatic error has not accidentally been induced by malapposition. In the case of vertical corneal laceration, the bites of these sutures may be short (Fig. 7-5B, left), about 1/2 mm, but in the case of a more oblique laceration, the sutures must have a longer bite (Fig. 7-5B, right), up to 1-1/2 mm to either side of the laceration, depending upon its obliquity. All sutures, however, should be placed as deeply as possible to Descemet's level to prevent a lambda-shaped (internally gaping) corneal closure. This internal gaping causes late flattening of the corneal curvature. This not only induces a thinner scar resulting in unnecessary optical errors, but also leaves a raw surface to which iris or lens or vitreous can adhere during healing, forming delayed anterior synechiae. When the wound is deeply and adequately closed, the anterior chamber is reformed by inserting carefully a 30-gauge needle through the incision so as not to damage uninvolved iris or lens, and the chamber is inflated with air to make certain that all iris, lens, and vitreous is free of the wound.

If the injury extends to the limbus at any point, a small peripheral iridectomy should be done at the lateral extent of the injury (Fig. 7-17). This will tend to prevent formation of an anterior synechia. Then, using 22-micron or 13-micron Ethilon suture on a GS-14 needle, a closely spaced, 1-mm running suture is placed at Descemet's level beginning at one end of the incision and running to the opposite end (Fig. 7-6, left). If the incision is irregular, x-shaped, or y-shaped, several running sutures, each closing a limb of the incision, may be used. In the case of an avulsing corneal injury, it may be necessary to close the apposed lacerations with interrupted sutures leaving the avulsed area open. This area can then be lightly marked with a trephine of appropriate size to cover the widest extent of the avulsion (Fig. 7-6, right). The same trephine is used to cut the corneal button from an eye-bank eye. The area outlined around the avulsion can then be excised freehand with microsurgical curved corneal scissors. The graft is sewn in place, using interrupted and continuous monofilament Ethilon suture, and the peripheral linear lacerations are repaired with interrupted or continuous sutures, as indicated.

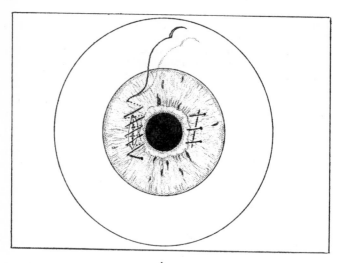

A

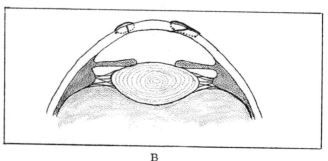

B

Fig. 7-5A. Diagrammatic representation of continuous suture (left) and interrupted sutures (right) for closure of linear corneal laceration.

Fig. 7-5B. Diagrammatic representation of closure of corneal lacerations: (left) vertical laceration closed with short bites (about 1/2 mm); (right) oblique laceration closed with longer bites (up to 1-1/2 mm).

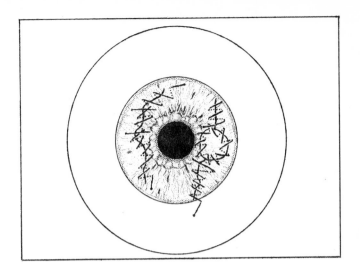

Fig. 7-6. (left) Irregular corneal laceration repaired with running
          suture; (right) avulsing corneal injury repaired with
          several running sutures. A corneal button from an eye-
          bank eye has been grafted in the avulsed area.

MANAGEMENT OF IRIS INCARCERATION: In the event of a simple
incarceration of the iris without laceration, iris may sometimes be
reposited by the use of a strong mydriatic or miotic and a little gentle external manipulation as soon as the patient is seen after injury.
Particularly if the penetrating injury is small and oblique, the incision may then close and the anterior chamber may reform spontaneously. Such a corneal laceration may not even require suturing. As
a general rule, a thorough examination of any penetrating corneal
injury, even without evident incarceration, should be made under
local or general anesthesia using the surgical microscope. Many
injuries will be found to be far greater in extent than suspected at
the first casual examination even when performed under slit-lamp
microscopy. The more peripheral the incarceration, the less likely
that it can be disengaged by the use of strong miotics or mydriatics.
Mechanical disengagement must then be performed and, since iris
manipulation is quite painful, should be done only under profound
local or general anesthesia. In the case of peripheral incarceration,
it is probably advisable to do an iridectomy and always to suture the
corneal laceration no matter how small it may appear. In the case
of very short lacerations, interrupted sutures should be used (see
Fig. 7-5A, right), tightly tied, and the flush-cut knot of the monofilament suture buried in corneal stroma. After resection or disengagement of the incarcerated iris, the anterior chamber should
be reformed with air. If air shows the iris to be disengaged, the air
should be partially or totally replaced with balanced salt solution so
that air pupillary block will not complicate the recovery. In the case
of the more peripheral simple iris incarcerations, the peripheral
iridectomy may be made peripheral to or in the incarcerated part

of the iris to prevent late reincarceration and synechiae. Mechanical separation of late synechiae may be possible with simple air injection using a 30-gauge needle through the closed corneal incision. If this does not succeed, however, the corneal incision must be partially reopened and resutured. The anterior chamber is again inflated with air or artificial aqueous humor so that the point of attachment of the incarceration can be seen and it can be verified that no suture is holding the incarceration in place. If so, the offending suture or sutures are removed and replaced so as not to engage the iris. An oblique corneal incision is then made about 2 mm anterior to the surgical limbus in clear cornea with a narrow, 1-mm keratome or a razor knife broken to a very narrow tip. A 1-mm spatula is inserted through this opening and the iris is carefully disengaged from the laceration incision. It is better to push the iris away from the sphincter toward the periphery rather than in the other direction, since too much pull peripherally may cause bleeding from the ciliary body or may produce an iridodialysis, or both. When the iris has been disengaged, air may be replaced with an acetylcholine solution to close the sphincter to a central position, pulling the iris down and away from the peripheral extent of the corneal laceration. If the inflammatory reaction of the eye can be suppressed effectively, continued miosis is preferable postoperatively to prevent reincarceration.

When the iris is badly lacerated, more extensive iridectomy is necessary to remove, surgically, traumatized and necrotic iris. This maneuver can be difficult through many primary corneal lacerations. If iris suture is to be employed to repair lacerated iris where sufficient iris remains to reform a stenopeic pupil, the average primary laceration incision is totally inadequate. The laceration must be extended (Fig. 7-7, A and B) by enlarging it with scissors so that an adequate exposure for iris repair can be obtained (Fig. 7-8) or the corneal laceration must be closed and a separate corneal or limbal incision made so that a more advantageous approach for surgical reconstruction is effected (Fig. 7-9). The use of the operating microscope and surgical slit lamp is extremely important to determine the extent of, and to repair, the iris laceration and incarceration and to perform more extensive reconstruction when there is posterior involvement of the lens and vitreous.

When lens is involved in anterior segment trauma which is blunt, non perforating or with only a small perforation without disruption, the lens should not be removed at the time of the primary repair but at a secondary procedure. If the lens has been badly lacerated, however, and the anterior capsule or the posterior capsule, or both, are ruptured, the corneal laceration should be repaired primarily (Fig. 7-10, A and B). A separate incision is then made (Fig. 7-10, A and B), and the lens material removed. Iris debridement and repair should be performed at the same procedure (Fig. 7-11). If vitreous has already presented or presents during the lens and iris procedures, anterior vitrectomy must be performed (Fig. 7-12, A and B). If an avulsing injury of the cornea accompanies this, a keratoplasty may also have to be performed.

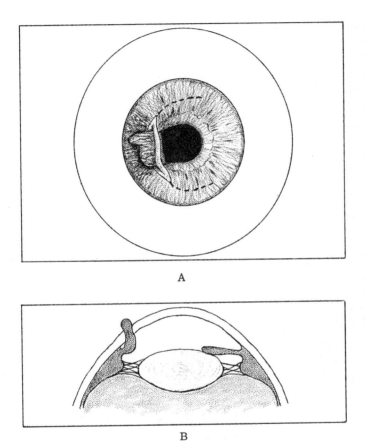

Fig. 7-7. A and B. Diagrammatic representation of iris incarcerated in the corneal wound. Dotted lines indicate proposed surgical incision to enlarge the wound.

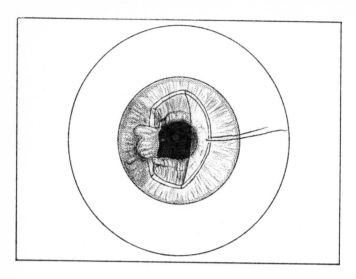

Fig. 7-8. Diagrammatic representation of surgical incision to enlarge the laceration to provide adequate exposure for repair.

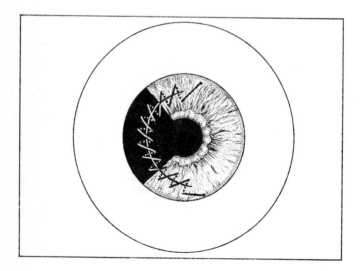

Fig. 7-9. Diagrammatic representation of corneal laceration and surgical incision closed with running suture. The necrotic iris has been excised.

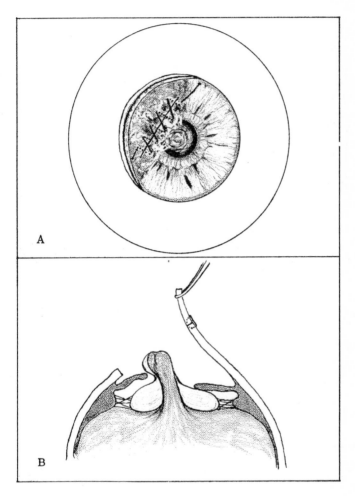

Fig. 7-10 A. Diagrammatic representation of primary closure of corneal laceration; separate limbal incision is made to remove lens material.

Fig. 7-10 B. Diagrammatic representation shows the cornea elevated; lens material and vitreous are shown in the anterior chamber.

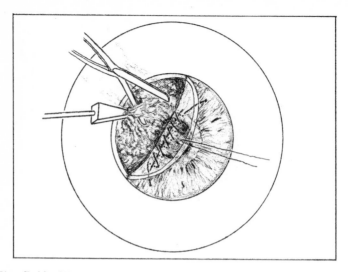

Fig. 7-11. Diagrammatic representation to show vitreous and lens
material being removed from the anterior chamber
using silastic Weck-Cel sponge and scissors.

It is becoming increasingly evident that simply to close a corneal
laceration and leave a badly disrupted anterior segment untreated
invites delayed intractable and later untreatable complications usually resulting in loss of vision or of the eye. Immediate reconstruction of the anterior segment offers a better opportunity to save such
badly damaged eyes but requires surgical instrumentation and skills
not currently available in every ophthalmic center, particularly in
the emergency room setting. If such a badly lacerated eye must be
simply closed because of untrained personnel or lack of microsurgical equipment, the patient should be transferred to an ophthalmic
surgical center within the first 48 hours after surgery so that the
eye may be reopened and the anterior segment primarily reconstructed. If the ciliary body is involved in a combined scleral corneal
laceration (Fig. 7-13), the eye has even less chance of survival and
there is an even greater necessity for painstaking repair and anterior segment reconstruction as a primary procedure. Excision of
traumatized and necrotic ciliary body by cyclectomy may be necessary to control bleeding which can persist from a lacerated ciliary
body (Fig. 7-14); vitrectomy must be performed and involved lens
and iris removed (Fig. 7-15, A and B). In all of these instances,
complete water-tight closure of the external laceration of the sclera
or cornea, or both, including, if necessary, corneal homograft,
should be done. This must be performed under microscopic magnification using microsurgical instrumentation and 22- or 13-micron
Ethilon suture in interrupted (Fig. 7-16) or continuous configuration.
Immediate postoperative care consists of suppression of infection
and inflammation. Bilateral patching should be used in the case of
peripheral lacerating injuries of the iris and of the ciliary body
where there is danger of bleeding. This should be combined with

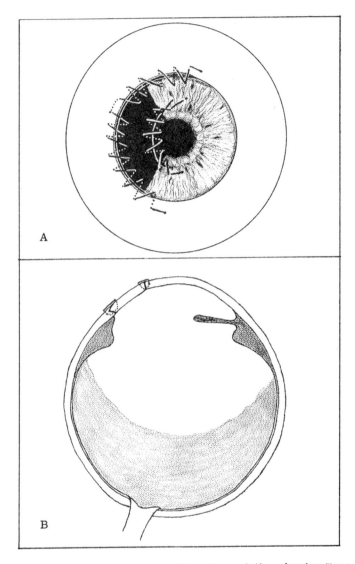

Fig. 7-12. A and B. Diagrammatic representation showing final stage of repair of laceration after corneal wound repair, iridectomy, lens extraction, and partial vitrectomy. (A) anterior view, and (B) cross-section.

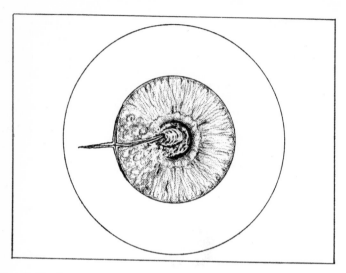

Fig. 7-13. Diagrammatic representation of corneoscleral laceration involving the ciliary body.

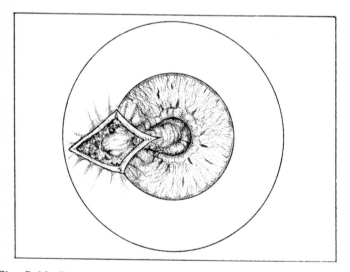

Fig. 7-14. Diagrammatic representation showing traumatized and
necrotic ciliary body in the wound.

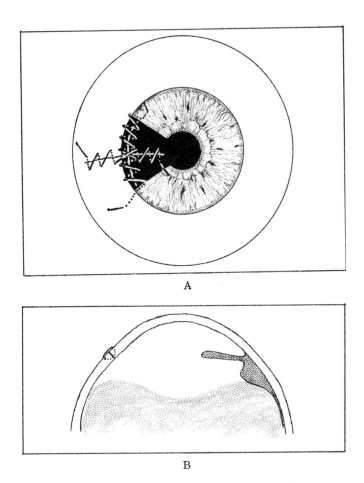

A

B

Fig. 7-15. A and B. Diagrammatic representation of corneoscleral laceration after iridectomy, cyclectomy, and lens extraction. (A) anterior view, and (B) cross-section.

sedation in the case of an unruly patient or a child. The healing eye should be followed biomicroscopically and keratometrically. Usually, no external dressing is necessary except for a shield during sleep and protective glasses during the day. The pupil should be maintained by mydriasis if there is continued inflammation, but miosis may be useful initially to keep the peripheral iris away from the freshly lacerated cornea. Topical steroids are indicated to control mild anterior inflammatory reaction but excessive or prolonged use may cause glaucoma or cataract. Centrally placed corneal sutures must not be removed for 3 to 6 months. Peripherally placed sutures may be removed in 1 to 3 months.

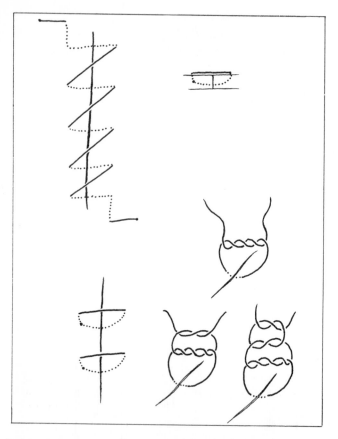

Fig. 7-16. Diagrammatic representation of suture configurations: (upper left) continuous suture; the dotted lines indicate suture placed deep in the cornea; (upper right) cross-section of interrupted suture, indicating depth of the suture, to close corneal laceration; (lower left) anterior view of interrupted sutures to close corneal laceration, dotted lines indicate suture placed deep in the cornea; (lower right) triple-knot configuration used with Ethilon sutures.

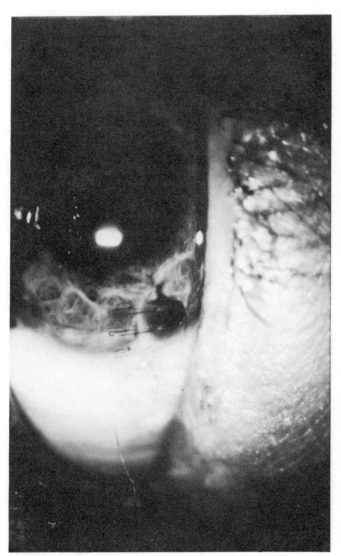

Fig. 7-17. A corneoscleral laceration after repair. Interrupted 10-0 Ethilon sutures and a small iridectomy are seen.

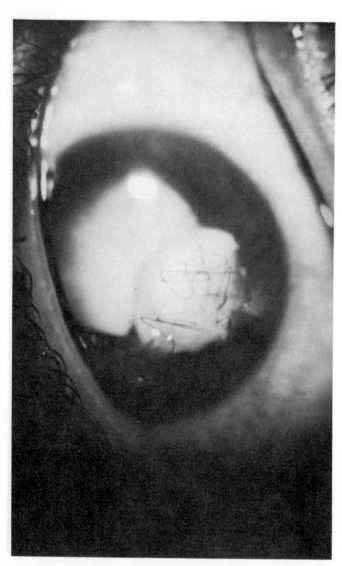

Fig. 7-18. Result of a poorly handled anterior segment injury. The corneal sutures are superficial and loose lens material fills up the anterior chamber.

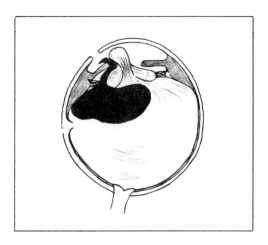

Fig. 7-19. Diagrammatic representation of a severely injured globe (cross-section); corneal and scleral wounds are present; lens material, vitreous and blood are shown in the anterior chamber; blood mixed with vitreous is shown in the vitreous cavity; the retina is torn at the site of the scleral wound.

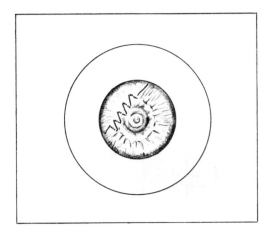

Fig. 7-20. Diagrammatic representation of primary closure of corneal laceration

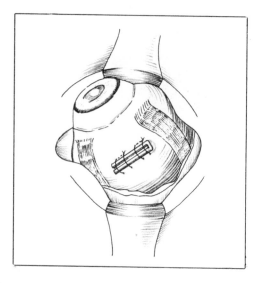

Fig. 7-21. Diagrammatic representation shows scleral buckle with silicone tire at the site of the repaired scleral wound.

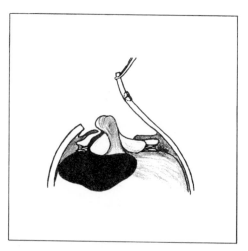

Fig. 7-22. Diagrammatic representation shows elevated cornea after closure of corneal laceration; a separate limbal incision is made to remove devitalized tissue (cross-section).

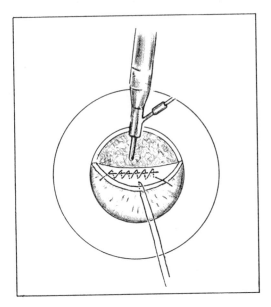

Fig. 7-23. Diagrammatic representation shows removal of devitalized tissue from the open eye using a vitrector.

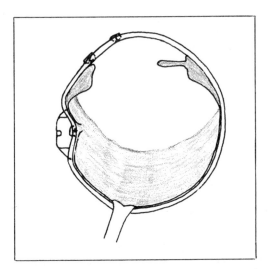

Fig. 7-24. Diagrammatic representation (cross-section) showing
the injured globe after repair of anterior and posterior
lacerations, corneal wound repair, iridectomy, lens
extraction, partial vitrectomy, scleral wound repair,
and scleral buckle.

EXTENSIVE INJURY OF THE EYEBALL

In severe or extensive injury to the eye, almost all structures of the eye, the cornea, the sclera, the lens, the uvea, the vitreous, and the retina can be involved. A recent concept, the so-called "primary repair of the severely injured globe" is considered an important development in the management of ocular trauma.

It seems to be an obsolete idea that trauma of the eyeball must be handled first by a so-called "anterior segment specialist" and later the case referred to a "retina man" or a "vitreous specialist" to repair posterior segment injuries. The ophthalmologist who handles trauma should care for the entire eye as soon as possible after the injury and all necessary repairs should be treated in one surgical session, if feasible.

Herewith the description of a hypothetic case: The eye sustained a perforating injury. A large corneal wound is present, the iris is torn, the lens is perforated and partly cataractous. A mixture of blood and vitreous is present in the anterior segment of the eye. Radiologic studies did not demonstrate a retained radiopaque intraocular foreign body. A double perforation, that is, an additional wound behind the ora serrata, is a very likely possibility (Fig. 7-19).

This case should be handled as follows: First, a water-tight closure of the corneal wound is achieved (Fig. 7-20). This is followed by a 360° peritomy. A search is made for the scleral wound. When it is found, it should be cleaned of tissue debris and closed with interrupted sutures. The area is sealed with cryocoagulation and a piece of silicone is sutured on the sclera to achieve a scleral buckle (Fig. 7-21). After completing this procedure, a separate, 180° limbal incision is made to remove traumatized, nonviable tissue from the anterior segment (Fig. 7-22).

A vitreous instrument (vitrector) is used to excise lens material mixed with blood and vitreous (Fig. 7-23). After the removal of all necrotic tissue, the remaining iris and the wound margins are carefully cleaned of vitreous debris and the surgical incision is closed with monofilament nylon sutures. The eyeball is then filled with physiologic solution and the intraocular pressure is restored to normal (Fig. 7-24).

The advantages of the primary repair are: (a) less post-traumatic complications, namely, less inflammation, less secondary glaucoma, less detached retina; (b) clear media; (c) better retinal function.

At present, no statistics are available to compare the primary repair approach with the multiple, step-by-step surgical repair; however, preliminary observations are in favor of the primary repair of the severely injured globe.

BIBLIOGRAPHY

1. Troutman, R. C. : The Operating Microscope in Ophthalmic Surgery. Trans Am Ophth Soc 63:335, 1965.

2. Troutman, R. C. : Microsurgery of the Eye, First Symp Ophth Microsurg Study Group, Tubingen, 1966. Adv Ophth 20:82, ed. Karger, Basel/New York, 1968.

3. Troutman, R. C. : Microsurgery of the Cornea. Bull NY Acad Med 45:53, 1969, No. 1.

4. Troutman, R. C. : Induced Astigmatism as a Result of Surgery. Trans First South African Ophth Symp, Johannesburg, South Africa, 1969.

5. Troutman, R. C. : Vitrectomy in Cataract and Corneal Surgery. Trans Pac Coast Oto-Ophth Soc, 1970, p. 157.

6. Troutman, R. C. : Ed. Microsurgery of Ocular Injuries. Third Int Symp Ophthal Microsurg Study Group, Merida, Yucatan, Mexico, 1970. Adv Ophth, Karger, Basel, 1972.

7. Faulborn, F. and Birnbaum, F. : Netzhautoperationen in verbindung mit der versorgung schwerer perforierender verletzungen. Klin Mbl Augenheilk 164:111, 1974.

8. Freeman, M. H. (Ed.): Ocular Trauma (in preparation).

9. Mackensen, G. and Faulborn, F. : Primary and secondary reconstruction of the eyeball after extensive lacerations. Ophth Surg 5:43, 1974.

CHAPTER 8

TRAUMA TO THE OPTIC NERVE

CONCUSSION INJURY OF THE OPTIC NERVE

The optic nerve of the eye is composed of approximately one million axons arising from the ganglion cell layer of the retina. The optic nerve is approximately 50 mm in length and is divisible into four components, an intraocular portion measuring about 0.7 mm, an orbital portion measuring approximately 33.0 mm, an intracanalicular portion measuring about 6.0 mm, and the intracranial portion measuring almost 10.00 mm.

Injury to the optic nerve is relatively common in concussion injuries. The optic nerve may be injured as a result of a frontal, frontotemporal, or orbital injury. There is usually some evidence of bruising around the eye, frequently accompanied by proptosis due to hemorrhage and edema within the orbit. Although a fracture of the skull in the frontal or temporal region is common, actual involvement of the optic canal is found in only a minority of cases. Occasionally, a fracture through the optic foramen with apparent compression of the nerve is evident, but such gross involvement of the nerve or actual tearing is uncommon. Indirect trauma to the optic nerve may account for immediate loss or pronounced reduction of vision and bitemporal hemianopsia. Immediate loss of vision represents a primary lesion involving the nerve and it is thought that the primary lesion is either a contusion necrosis or an actual tear. Contusion necrosis is thought to occur within one millisecond from the time of trauma.

The optic nerve head picture remains normal with the exception of a few retinal hemorrhages. Any improvement in vision, either partial or complete, commences within a few days and reaches its maximum improvement in about three weeks, at which time the optic nerve becomes pale. The secondary effects of indirect trauma to the optic nerve or chiasm may result from edema which can be caused either by the contusion itself or by hypoxia. It is thought also that the necrosis may be induced by systemic circulatory failure or by the local compression of vessels. If the loss of vision occurred at the moment of impact, it is unlikely that therapy would increase the chances of improving or restoring vision. If it can be established that there was vision after the impact, even if only for a few minutes, the lesion or lesions responsible for the loss of vision are secondary. In these cases, emergency surgical intervention such as surgical removal of the roof of the optic canal may have a beneficial effect.

In the affected eye, the pupil does not react or reacts very poorly to direct light. If the oculomotor nerve is intact, light presented to the contralateral eye will cause a brisk contraction of the pupil of the

affected eye, but light presented to the affected eye will not cause
constriction of the opposite pupil. These consensual reactions serve
to distinguish between optic nerve and oculomotor nerve injury as a
cause of the nonreacting pupil. If the eye itself is undamaged and the
optic fundus is normal, a diagnosis of optic nerve or chiasmal injury can be established.

When the optic nerve lesion is complete, even though initially the
optic disc looks normal, pallor gradually develops and is usually
unequivocal within three to six weeks. Once these changes are established and the patient has no light perception, permanent blindness is the rule. However, partial injuries to the optic nerve are
more common and in these circumstances one should not reach an
adverse prognosis too hastily. Even slight evidence of recovery, as
judged by perception of light or reaction of the pupil within the first
48 hours, can be followed by a marked degree of recovery and improvement may continue for several months. If the lesion is partial,
the most common visual field defect is in the inferior quadrants.

Traumatic hemorrhages into the optic nerve sheath are probably not
very common and may be subdural or subarachnoid in type. It is
usually difficult to differentiate between the two types. Funduscopic
appearance or traumatic hemorrhages into the optic nerve sheath
may show papilledema and hemorrhages around the optic disc. The
retinal arteries are normal. All these changes are believed to be
caused by increased pressure around the optic nerve.

An injury to the optic chiasm may occur when a fracture crosses
the region of the stella turcica and the optic chiasm may also be
torn by severe injury (gunshot wound through the skull close to the
chiasmal area). A pure chiasmal lesion produces a bitemporal
hemianopsia, but more often the chiasmal lesion is combined with
a more obvious optic nerve injury on one side.

In considering the differential diagnosis of loss of vision following
trauma, one must consider, in addition to direct trauma to the optic nerve, the pressure caused by lid swelling, corneal damage, and
blood or foreign material inside the eye. The blood may be in the
form of hyphema or a vitreous hemorrhage. Other considerations
include traumatic cataract, luxation of the lens, central retinal artery or vein occlusion, traumatic retinal edema and hemorrhages,
retinal detachment, an episode of acute angle-closure glaucoma,
hysteria, and malingering.

RUPTURE AND EVULSION OF THE OPTIC NERVE

The most common cause of rupture and evulsion of the optic nerve
is a penetrating injury of the orbit. It may result also from severe
direct concussion of the globe. Very often such an injury is associated with gross intraocular hemorrhage and intraocular damage.
Rupture of the optic nerve can be partial or complete. Pathologic
examination of these cases show an irregular transverse tear at the
level of the termination of Bruch's elastic lamina.

The ophthalmoscopic appearance of a complete rupture reveals partial or complete absence of retinal vessels. The optic disc appears as a bottomless pit set in a background in which there are contusion changes.

The vision is gravely impaired in case of a partial rupture of the nerve. In complete rupture of the nerve, vision loss is complete and irreversible. There is no effective treatment in these cases.

BIBLIOGRAPHY

1. Cogan, D. G. : Neurology of the Visual System. Charles C Thomas, Springfield, Ill. , 1966.

2. Duke-Elder, S. : System of Ophthalmology, Vol. XIV. Injuries. Mosby, St. Louis, 1972.

3. Walsh, F. B. : Pathological-clinical correlations. 1. Indirect trauma to the optic nerves and chiasm. Invest Ophthal 5:433, 1966.

4. Walsh, F. B. and Hoyt, W. F. : Clinical Neuro-ophthalmology, 3rd Ed. Williams and Wilkins Company, Baltimore, 1969.

CHAPTER 9

TRAUMA OF THE EYELIDS, ORBIT, AND ADNEXA

INTRODUCTION

The ophthalmic surgeon should be a member of the emergency team when facial injuries occur. The failure to recognize serious ocular injuries at the time of initial treatment may cause loss of vision.

Life-saving measures have priority and the ophthalmologist must await the treatment of shock and the establishment of an airway and respiratory function before examining the patient who is seriously injured. The team approach in the operative treatment of serious trauma shortens the time required for surgical repair and assures that the best final result is attained under the circumstances. When trauma is confined to the lids and adnexa, the ophthalmologist may undertake the repair immediately.

TYPES OF INJURIES

LACERATING INJURIES: These injuries are commonly caused by the sharp edges of glass or metal. They are frequently encountered in automobile accidents. No loss of tissue is expected. The edges of the wound usually lie in good apposition, with edema occasionally causing some slight displacement. Adjacent to the lacerated areas may be heavily abraded skin surfaces ingrained with road dirt or grease. These must be thoroughly scrubbed to prevent a tatooing which is very difficult to treat and requires dermabrasion after complete healing has taken place. A retained foreign body which may be in the depths of the wound may be irrigated from the wound during preparation for surgery or may be palpated and removed. In the operating room, exploration of the extent of the wound by disruption reveals the true extent of the injury. Penetrating wounds may show only a small wound of entry but must be carefully explored. Many cases have been reported of cranial cavity entry with major central nervous system complications and, in a personally observed case, such an injury has caused death. Umbrella tips, automobile aerials, and sharp sticks are common offenders. [1]

Puncture wounds of the lids caused by sharp-tipped objects, especially metal-tipped darts, may conceal a perforating injury of the globe. Even if the site of lid puncture seems remote, a visual acuity and careful indirect ophthalmoscopy may reveal a perforating injury of the globe. [2]

DISRUPTION AND PARTIAL AVULSION: When a direct blow to the eye is sufficiently violent to tear the lid, the globe underneath is rarely unscathed and ruptures of the posterior globe must be considered. The structures of the ruptured lid are irregular but are easily reconstructed since no fragments are avulsed.

When avulsion of the lid occurs by a hook or finger from beneath the lid, it is usually medial to the punctum (Fig. 9-1). The tear is usually vertical and medial to the tarsus, then turns abruptly horizontally through the upper cul-de-sac above the tarsus, these being the structurally weaker areas. A glancing blow on the nasal side can partially avulse either or both lids at a point between the medial canthus and the puncta. All medially located lacerations or avulsions must be carefully inspected to determine the integrity of the lacrimal drainage apparatus. An attempt must always be made to repair the canaliculi but the loss of function of only one canaliculus may not affect tear drainage. [3]

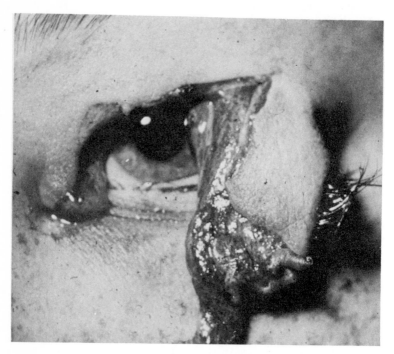

Fig. 9-1. Partial avulsion of lid

Total avulsion of either or both lids is rare. However, the number of reported human and animal bites of the lids is sufficient to warrant the search for the portion of lid that is missing to use it in the repair. [4] The survival of at least the tarsal structures may be of great assistance in the reconstruction and avoids the use of substitutes (nasal cartilage, septum, or ear cartilage).

FRACTURES: Fractures of the bony substructures must be searched for with a gloved finger in the depth of the wound and with x-rays. In addition to the expected blow-out fractures of the floor and medial wall, rim fractures above and below may cause restriction in motility of the globe as well as the lid (Figs. 9-2 and 9-3). (One case of blow-out fracture of the roof of the orbit has been reported.[5]) In addition to plain films, tomography and hypocyloidal tomography should be ordered to identify the site and extent of the fracture. It is at this time that a request is made for consultation with the appropriate specialist (plastic surgeon, oral surgeon, otolaryngologist, neurosurgeon) so that evaluation and plans for treatment can be made jointly.

A systematic method of evaluation of the injuries should be followed:

1. If the state of consciousness allows, measure the visual acuity using a reading card for the younger patient and a Snellen chart or finger counting at 20 feet for the older individual, with correction if available. The medical-legal implications cannot be overemphasized.

2. Inspect the wounds using intense illumination and determine immediately if the globe is involved. Diagnostic features of laceration and rupture of the globe are described in Chapters V and VI.

3. Irrigate the wound depths freely. Use sterile gloves and pad to determine if the wounds involve bone (compound fractures), palpate for crepitation, fragments of loose bone, and foreign bodies. Identify the missing areas of lid tissue and the layers involved. Determine also if the lacrimal structure or ocular muscles are involved.

TREATMENT: Administration of tetanus antitoxin or tetanus toxoid should be considered at the time of admission to the hospital or emergency room. The use of preventive antibiotic therapy in lid wounds is not recommended, but intense antibiotic therapy is required in cases of orbito-cranial wounds.

If the area of injury is severely edematous with tensed, stretched tissues, it may be preferable to use a sterile antiseptic dressing and delay therapy for 12 hours. The concept of early repair is still valid when the tissues can be handled easily and swelling will not cause excessive suture tension.

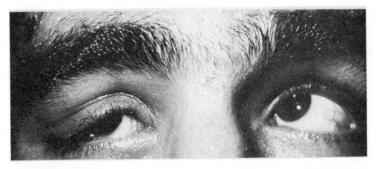

Fig. 9-2. Rim fracture causing restriction of motility

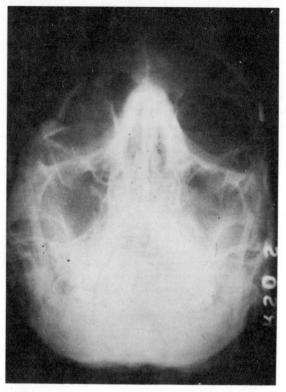

Fig. 9-3. X-ray picture of a rim fracture causing restriction of
    motility

SURGICAL TREATMENT: General anesthesia is preferred if available and if the patient's condition is good. The length of time required for the repair cannot be predicted and the surgeon is not
rushed by the limitations of local anesthesia. If local anesthesia is
selected, Xylocaine or Carbacaine 1% without hyaluronidase may be
used. If epinephrine is added, a dilution of 1/200 thousand is preferable to 1/100 thousand. If a large amount of agent is used, a
toxic dose may be approached, e. g. , 200 cc of 2% Xylocaine de-
livers 400 mgs of anesthetic agent. This amount may affect the dis-
eased myocardium of an elderly patient or cause toxic effects to the
cerebrum resulting in disorientation. If the local anesthesia must be
reinforced, 1/2% solution of Xylocaine is effective without the likelihood of approaching a toxic level.

Because the sensory apparatus for pain is derived from branches of
the trigeminal nerve, the lids and areas surrounding the orbit can
be blocked by injections which penetrate the orbital septum at the
site of exit of the various branches of the nerve (Figs. 9-4A and

9-4B). In addition, the infraorbital foramen may be blocked by entering the skin of the cheek approximately 10 mm from the naris and in line with the supraorbital notch. The opening for the foramen is reached by sliding the needle along the groove superiorly toward the orbital rim until the needle point is locked into the foramen. At this point, the patient may complain of pain in his teeth. An injection of a 1/4 to 1/2 cc Xylocaine quickly anesthetizes a major part of the lower lid. Infiltration of lid, especially when there has been fragmentation of the lid border and partial avulsion of the lid itself, sometimes is ineffective.

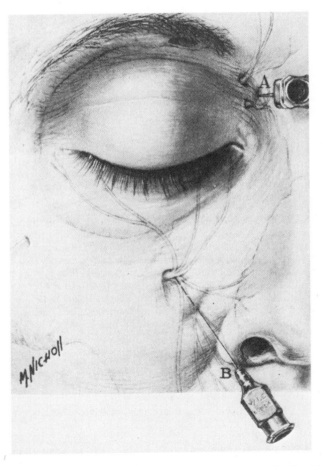

Fig. 9-4A. Anesthesia of the (a) supratrochlear and (b) infratrochlear nerves. (Reprinted with the permission of the publisher and the author.) Callahan, A.: Reconstructive surgery of the eyelids and ocular adnexa. Aesculapius Pub. Co., Birmingham.

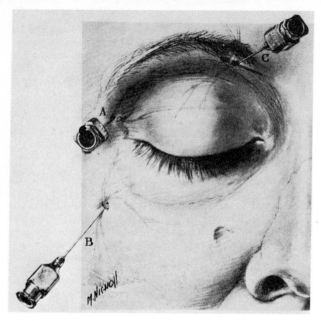

Fig. 9-4B. Anesthesia of the (a) lacrymal, (b) zygomatico-facial,
(c) supraorbital nerves. (Reprinted with the permission
of the publisher and the author.) Callahan, A. : Reconstructive surgery of the eyelids and ocular adnexa.
Aesculapius Pub. Co. , Birmingham.

PREPARATION: Betadine is extremely effective and useful to clean
the wound and the surrounding area. [7] It has been found to be moderately irritating to the eye but has never caused damage to the
globe. One author has reported Betadine in half-strength to be an
effective irrigant for the cul-de-sac. After anesthesia has been administered, repeated minute inspections of the wound are carried out
to the extent that a microscope may be brought into use to identify
the severed ends of the canaliculi. The time spent arranging the
jigsaw puzzle of lid lacerations is never wasted. After the bleeding
has been curtailed and the edges fitted together it may become apparent for the first time that there is a partial avulsion of a lid border or that a lid which was previously thought to have been badly
damaged has, in fact, all of its parts and can be easily repaired with
simple suturing.

Lid tissues have remarkable vitality; and extensive debridement is
not necessary.

LACERATIONS: Simple lacerations in line with the orbicularis fibers should be closed with 6-0 or 7-0 silk; deep gut sutures are not
necessary since the lines of tension do not predispose towards gaping of the wound. The tissue involved in any vertical wound, especially if the wound extends to the brow above or below to the malar
area, is capable of shrinkage and so provisions should be made for

meticulous closure of the wound with possible Z-plasty (Figs. 9-5, 9-6, and 9-7) to prevent contraction.

The injury which extends from the brow and lacerates the lid and its border, lacerates also the lower lid and its border and extends over the malar area is most likely to lead to a retraction and notching of the lids (Fig. 9-8A). The closure of through-and-through lacerations of the lid is dependent on the exact alignment of the anterior and posterior lid borders (Fig. 9-8B). The use of 6-0 or 7-0 silk on very sharp needles has made it possible for both an anterior and posterior aligning suture to be inserted through the lid borders. In addition, a suture may be placed through the gray line (Fig. 9-9). The lashes are the most important landmark in aligning lid borders. If lash continuity is precise it is of very little consequence if the posterior border shows a small notch. The central gray line suture is sufficient to keep the lid border in tight apposition. All the sutures placed in the fibrous tissues of the tarsus can take a good purchase and, once tied, serve well to maintain the continuity of the lid curve. Once the anterior aligning suture is placed and the surgeon's tie is drawn up, the lid can be tensioned, the assistant keeping the aligning suture taut (Fig. 9-10). The inferior extent of the wound in the culde-sac is isolated and picked up on a sharp hook. The wound may be closed with an interrupted or running 6-0 plain suture, the inferior border of the tarsus serving as an additional landmark for alignment. A running or interrupted gut suture will serve as satisfactorily as a running externalized nylon suture. In some instances, it has been necessary to leave nylon in the wound because it has broken off, especially when 6-0 nylon is put under very great tension when attempting its removal. Nonabsorbable running sutures placed in subcutaneous tissues must be drawn very tightly so that they can cut through eventually and be removed more easily. The skin is then closed with interrupted silk and the three aligning sutures are tied. If the wound extends through the orbital area into the malar or frontal area, the linear wound must be broken by at least one Z-plasty to prevent the extreme end of the wound from serving as an anchor upon which the scar contracts.

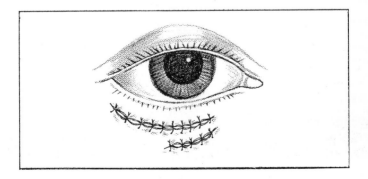

Fig. 9-5. Closure of laceration parallel to the orbicularis muscle

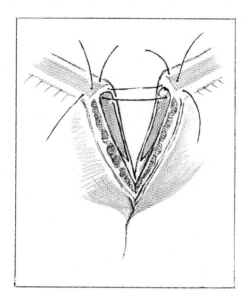

Fig. 9-6. Closure of vertical lacerations; marginal aligning sutures are shown.

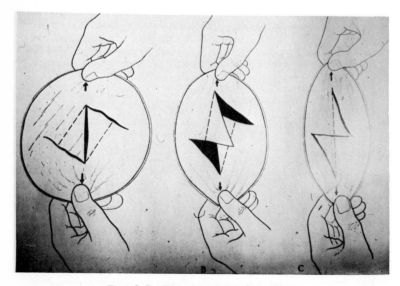

Fig. 9-7. The principle of Z-plasty

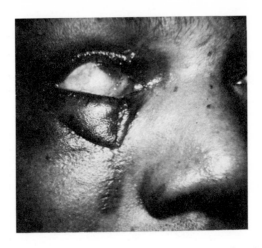

Fig. 9-8A. Vertical laceration causing notching and retraction of the lower lid.

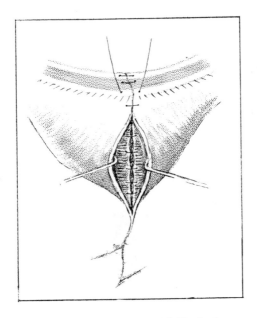

Fig. 9-8B. Closure with Z-plasty

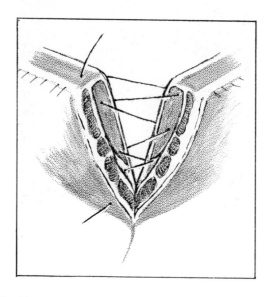

Fig. 9-9A. Closure of vertical laceration with 6-0 nylon running sutures.

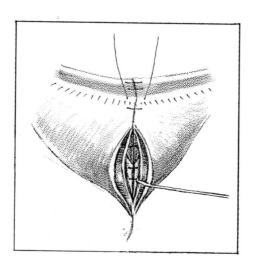

Fig. 9-9B. Closure of vertical laceration with interrupted gut sutures in the tarsus.

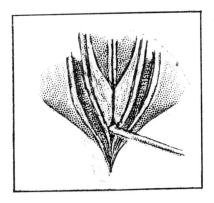

Fig. 9-10. The inferior extent of the wound picked up on sharp hook and closure with interrupted gut sutures.

PARTIAL AVULSIONS: The partially avulsed lid requires (Figs. 9-1 and 9-11), in addition to the meticulous closure, as described in simple lacerations, a mattress suture which is inserted through the sturdy tarsus and along the periosteum above the level of the insertion of the canthal ligament out through the skin. This 4-0 silk suture is drawn up and tied after the lid borders have been aligned (Fig. 9-12) and the deep gut sutures have been tied. It is, however, the first suture to be inserted and it is adjusted so that, when it is tensioned prior to any other suturing, the lid borders are in good alignment. The suture is loosened and the lid is turned back. The conjunctival cul-de-sac is identified and brought forward on 2 traction sutures. The tissue immediately anterior to the superior cul-de-sac conjunctiva consists of Mueller's muscle and if one proceeds sufficiently, superiorly, one reaches the beginning of the expansion of levator muscle. In repairing the partially avulsed lid it is important that the conjunctiva and Mueller's muscle be carefully joined. The tissues immediately anterior to Mueller's muscle must be united with the corresponding layer in the upper lid since, at the point of the superior border of the tarsus, the forward extension of the levator muscle interdigitates with the orbicularis. An attempt must always be made to reestablish the integrity of the canaliculus and, in fact, this effort may be helpful in realigning the lid borders. One of the more successful methods has been the use of the Worst pigtail probe[6] (Fig. 9-13A). Many modifications have been described including the formation of a French eye or a drill hole in the end of the probe (Fig. 9-13B). Many methods have been described for passing a stent tubing through the lacerated canaliculus. A useful method to pass the polyethylene tubing is described by Werb (Fig. 9-14). The polyethylene tubing is passed in a circle so that the two open ends appear in the palpebral fissure. One end is then stretched and passed into the opposite lumen. Heat is applied gently with the cau-

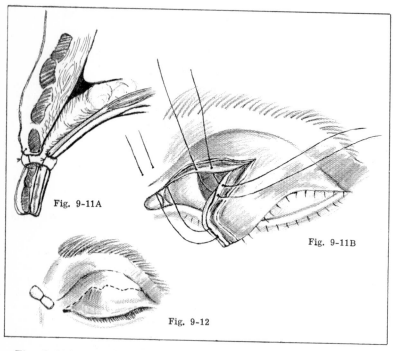

Fig. 9-11A.

Fig. 9-11B.

Fig. 9-12.

Fig. 9-11A. Cross-section indicating two-layer closure of partially
          avulsed lid.
Fig. 9-11B. Placing of mattress tension suture in the wound.
Fig. 9-12.   Lid repaired with tension suture tied over gauze peg.

tery held at a small distance from the tubing to prevent burning
which causes the adherence of the inner tube to the outer tube. The
tubing is then rotated into the punctum so that the broken loop of
polyethylene tubing lies between the two puncta in the palpebral fissure. If the punctum and the portion of the canaliculus have been
totally avulsed, it may be wiser to incise the posterior wall of the
canaliculus and suture the mucous membrane lining of the canaliculus to the conjunctiva, forming a gutter (Fig. 9-15).

A special bodkin with a swagged nylon suture or the Worst pigtail
probe with a perforated tip is passed through the punctum of the less
obstructed canaliculus into the dacryocystorrhinostomy opening. The
free end of the nylon suture is passed through the tubing which has a
1.5 mm outside diameter and a thread, then clamp through the tubing with a hemostat. The end of the tube closer to the needle, the
end which is to enter the punctum, is stretched, causing it to taper
and break. The excess polyethylene tubing is removed by slitting one

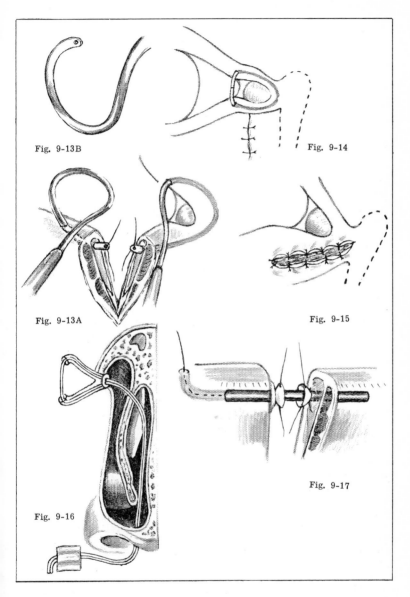

Fig. 9-13B

Fig. 9-14

Fig. 9-13A

Fig. 9-15

Fig. 9-16

Fig. 9-17

Fig. 9-13A. Pigtail probes introduced into the canaliculi.
Fig. 9-13B. Drill hole at the tip of pigtail probe.
Fig. 9-14. Continuous polyethylene strand for lacerated canaliculus.
Fig. 9-15. Canaliculus converted to drainage gutter.
Fig. 9-16. Position of polyethylene tubing after the method of Werb.
Fig. 9-17. Veir's canaliculus rod in place, 9-0 or 10-0 nylon in membranous canaliculus.

end and pulling it against the nylon thread which acts as a cutting edge. The tapered end is lubricated and pulled gently into the canaliculus; this procedure is repeated for the opposite canaliculus. Both ends of the tubing are passed through the bony ostium, into the nasal passage, out through the nostril, and fastened to the face with tape (Fig. 9-16).

A few days later, a collar may be slipped over the two ends of the tubing, into the nasal passage,adjusting the loop by raising the collar for a smaller loop, allowing it to remain lower for a larger loop. In the case of a fresh laceration, the tubing must be kept in place for six to eight weeks.

If the sac itself has been avulsed or destroyed it may be necessary to use the double-tube Werb technique in a dacryocystorrhinostomy ostium, using the nasal mucosal flap as the anterior and posterior walls of the passageway, suturing the walls to the remnant of the common canaliculus or the common canaliculus area.

An extremely useful device based on a completely different principle is the Veir's canaliculus rod (Ethicon) which is attached to a 4-0 single-armed suture. The rod is placed in a horizontal portion of the canaliculus and serves as a stent for the repair. The cuff of the canaliculus around the rod is closed with a very fine suture. The rod is then maintained in position by placing a 4-0 silk suture bite in the skin. This technique holds the distal end of the rod firmly against the vertical portion of the canaliculus (Fig. 9-17). While attempting to repair a torn canaliculus it is imperative that no damage be done to the canaliculus in the other lid.

If both canaliculi have been lacerated, the repair may be combined with a dacryocystorrhinostomy or a circular polyethylene tube using the technique of Werb.

If there is total avulsion of the lid or lids, every effort must be made to locate the avulsed tissue. If the avulsed lid is found, it is placed in a sterile pad moistened with a dilute antibiotic solution and utilized as a free composite graft, hoping that the graft will take in the excellent vascular bed. Should there be an avulsion with total loss of tissue, the conjunctiva of the cul-de-sac down to the limbus should be completely mobilized. The opposite lid is prepared with a compound pedicle flap. It is possible to block the lids and areas surrounding the orbit by using injections which penetrate the orbital septum at the site of exit of the various branches of the ophthalmic division (see Fig. 9-4).

TOTAL AVULSION: Avulsed Portion Available for Replacement: When the avulsed portion of the lid has been properly oriented with regard to the defect, the component layers of the recipient areas are identified by placing traction sutures on conjunctiva dissected in the cul-de-sac above or below. In the upper lid, as previously described, pulling down on the traction sutures helps to identify the levator muscle immediately anterior to this conjunctival layer. In the case of avulsion of the lower lid, the extension of the inferior rectus muscle need not be sutured through the orbitalis fascia into the lid as this technique only permits the lid to be lowered. It has not been apparent that the eye functions less well if the lower lid does not move down equally well as the fellow lid.

The superior border of the conjunctiva and tarsus of the avulsed portion is joined with a pull-out suture or with a running 5-0 or 6-0 chromic suture with bites taken very closely together to insure a firm union. The aligning sutures are placed on either end of the avulsed portion, as they would for a laceration, to line up the fragment with the recipient portions of the lid. The running gut suture may now be placed in the vertical or oblique portions of the avulsed lid utilizing either the buried suture through the tarsus with the double knot tied near the superior fornix or a pull-out nylon suture. The aligning sutures are then drawn up and tied and the skin closed with running suture in the horizontal portion of the wound and interrupted sutures in the vertical portion.

Through-and-through mattress sutures near the borders of the lid with pegs on the skin surface may be used to reduce the tension on the margin of the lids (see Fig. 9-12).

The repair of the canaliculi is carried out as described above. When the lacerations are multiple and there is some question regarding the loss of tissue, it is necessary that the final arrangement of tissues be made so that there is no tension on the small flap. The loss of anterior layer can be replaced immediately by full-thickness skin grafts from the opposite upper lid or from behind the ear.

AVULSION COMPOUND PEDICLE FLAP FOR REPAIR OF AVULSED SITE: If both lids are avulsed, the conjunctiva above and below should be thoroughly mobilized (down to the limbus, if necessary) and the edges of the conjunctiva sutured together to provide a closed, protective envelope. A full-thickness graft from behind the ear or, preferably, from the opposite upper lid tissue, if available, is placed over the closed conjunctival wound to provide an outer layer covering. This is an emergency treatment which will be modified later to provide a more acceptable cosmetic and visual result. Should a coloboma secondary to trauma exist in the upper lid, the method of Cutler and Beard described in 1955 may be used.[9]

An incision is made at the inferior border of the tarsus, 1/3 less in width than the coloboma in the upper lid. The vertical incisions are made into the inferior cul-de-sac at either end of the horizontal incision. These through-and-through incisions form a compound pedicle flap consisting of skin, orbicularis, and conjunctiva. The flap is advanced beneath the bridge, which includes the lid border and the marginal arcade, into the coloboma and is sutured using a nylon pull-out suture in the advancing edge of the flap or interrupted 5-0 or 6-0 plain gut sutures. The vertical portions are locked in place at the upper lid border with 5-0 or 6-0 gut sutures and the skin is sutured in place with 6-0 or 7-0 silk. At the end of eight to ten weeks, the pedicle flap is severed, allowing an excess in the upper lid, and the wound edges in the lower lid are trimmed to provide fresh wound surfaces. The skin and conjunctival flaps are sutured to their respective layers in the lower lid.

A similar procedure is performed if there is a coloboma in the lower lid, with the incision being made in the tarsus, if the inferior lid coloboma is shallow. (Five to 6 mm of the tarsus of the upper lid may be used to reconstruct tarsus of the lower lid.) If the defect is extensive and deep, the incision is made at the superior border of the tarsus and the entire compound pedicle flap (1/3 less in width than the defect below) is advanced beneath the tarsal margin of the upper lid and into the defect below. A closure similar to that described above is utilized. When the pedicle flap is severed eight to ten weeks later, the convexity is toward the upper lid, allowing for excess tissue which can be trimmed at a later date.

LACRIMAL SYSTEM: Lacerations - Canaliculi ... Repairs of the canaliculi have already been described.

DESTRUCTION OF THE LACRIMAL SAC: If the lacrimal sac has been lacerated or the two canaliculi severed from the body of the sac, thus destroying the common canaliculus and causing lack of drainage, it is necessary that an attempt be made by the use of polyethylene or teflon tubing to reestablish drainage by means of a dacryocystorrhinostomy according to the method of Werb. Werb has shown that the placement of the double tubing into the vertical portion of the lacrimal canal does not provide as effective drainage as when the ostium is made through the lacrimal sac fossa into the nose anterior to the superior concha (see Fig. 9-16).

Lacerations through the upper lid that involve the lacrimal gland and that separate the palpebral portion of the gland from the orbital portion of the gland, do not necessarily cause a dry eye since the glands of the fornix may very well provide sufficient lubrication for the globe. There is no method for reestablishing lacrimal gland secretion.

FRACTURES OF THE ORBIT: When the bony framework of the globe absorbs the major part of the trauma, the globe is usually preserved. The types of fractures range from the pure blow-out of the floor, which has been so adequately described, to extensive multiple comminuted and compounded fractures of frontal, zygomatic maxillary bones. It is in the area of fractures that the greatest overlap of subspecialty responsibility occurs. The pure blow-out fracture in which the stability of the facial frame is undisturbed and trauma is limited to the orbit, may be confined to the ophthalmology service. This is true also of fracture of the ethmoid with its accompanying emphysema which is demonstrated easily in x-ray films. Dislocations and fractures of the zygoma and fractures of the roof and superior rim of the orbit along with major maxillary and nasal dislocations require the combined efforts of the surgical subspecialties.

"PURE BLOW-OUT FRACTURE": When a blow to the orbit is caused by an object whose major circumference is larger than the aperture of the orbit, the portion which impinges on the globe may cause sufficient compression of the orbital contents to fracture a portion of the floor or the ethmoid sinuses without any disturbance to the sturdy rim structures. (Trauma of such a type may be caused by a baseball, a fist, a child's buttock, or a basketball.) The history of a blow, followed by dizziness, nausea, and sudden vomiting, sudden onset of numbness of the lip on the side of the injury, and double vision have all been described extensively. There may be little or no ecchymosis or, in contrast, there may be a marked orbital hemorrhage with edema and ecchymosis of the lids and subconjunctival hemorrhage. Subcutaneous crepitation may be present at injury or may occur subsequent to the injury if the patient tries to clear his nose by blowing, thus forcing air through the ruptured ethmoid walls into the orbit. A significant symptom is pain on the injured side when attempting to look up or down. Exploration in these cases reveals an impingement of a spicula of bone on the inferior rectus muscle or an entrapment by a splinter fracture. Standard Waters views and lateral views are used and should be supplemented by special views including tomography to determine the true extent of the fracture. In addition, the traction test may be useful to determine the entrapment of the inferior rectus or the medial rectus muscle. Also, traction may be curative in some cases where the muscle can be teased free from a small fracture. In order to do an adequate traction test, local anesthesia and the cooperation of the patient in looking up with both eyes is necessary. The test must be done with an adequate grasp of the insertion of the inferior rectus muscle in addition to the grasp at the limbus. Despite radiologic findings of a blow-out fracture, surgical intervention is not indicated unless the restriction in motility causing diplopia persists for a week to ten days and the traction test remains positive. In some instances, when the pain is severe on attempted elevation, earlier intervention may be indicated. It is certainly not necessary to treat this injury as an emergency and, on the contrary, a delay of several days with enzyme or steroid therapy, or both, by mouth, may allow sufficient time for all symptoms to disappear and thus eliminate the need for surgery. Any delay in surgery will allow absorption of much of the hemorrhage and edema, providing increased working space and better identification of tissues. The prognosis of cases in which surgery has been delayed for ten days to two weeks is not altered. The long-term follow-up of cases operated indicates that approximately 20% retain the diplopia and 10% have enophthalmos despite the use of an implant.

Long-term follow-ups in cases which have not been operated show that in the young individual an appropriate adjustment is made to the minimal diplopia in upward gaze and the patient continues to function well. The incidence of enophthalmos increases to over 20% and the cosmetic deformity is tolerated in most instances (Figs. 9-18 and 9-19).

THERMAL BURNS OF THE LIDS: Thermal burns of the lids, when limited in extent (such as cigarette ash or small bits of molten metal) do not require specific therapy since the injury is not sufficiently extensive to cause deformities of the lid or damage to the

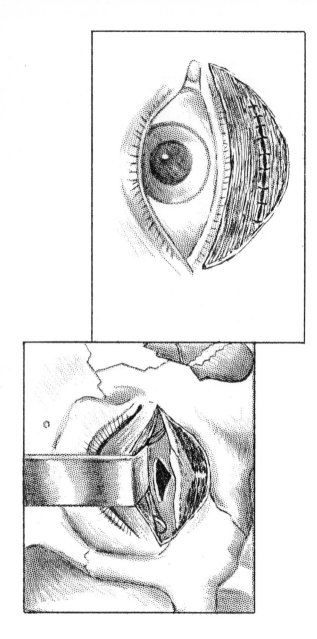

Fig. 9-18. Typical fracture site
Fig. 9-19. Site of incision. The two-plane approach and the repair

globe. When, as is common, the burns are extensive and include the face and body, the primary physician should be the plastic surgeon, with consultation with the ophthalmologist.

CHEMICAL BURNS: Chemical burns are an emergency and require immediate therapy. The most useful and immediately available therapy is extensive showering, as described by Bromberg. The hydrotherapy (using a hose or shower) of the patient who has received chemical burns of the face and lids reduces the need for extensive grafting and has been shown to reduce the extent of third-degree chemical burns.

FOREIGN BODIES IN THE ORBIT: The mere presence of metallic foreign bodies in the orbit does not necessarily require surgical intervention. Large objects which interfere mechanically with the motility of the globe must be removed. Plastic material such as methyl-methacrylate and lead particles of small size may be left safely if they do not interfere mechanically with movement of the globe. Occasionally, a study of the eye will reveal increasing edema of the retina. When the x-ray studies indicate the foreign body is in close proximity to the scleral wall, it may be necessary to remove the foreign body because of its irritating nature.

The case shown (Fig. 9-20) is one in which a fragment of a 22-calibre lead bullet was resting on the sclera at the macular area and causing increasing edema during the week following the injury.

The presence of wood fragments in the orbit may lead to chronic infection and fistulization. Therefore, during the initial repair of the injury, the surgeon must search carefully for such fragments and remove them with an exploratory incision, if necessary.

The standard technique for the removal of orbiral foreign bodies which lie behind the equator of the globe is the temporal or lateral orbitotomy (modified Kronlein approach), which provides excellent exposure.

For foreign bodies which may be lodged anterior to the equator of the globe, an anterior approach is satisfactory.

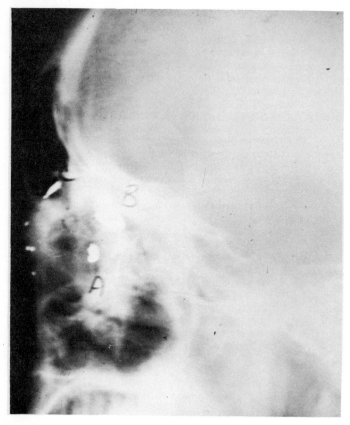

Fig. 9-20. Foreign body, (lead) bullet fragment resting on the posterior aspect of the sclera.

BIBLIOGRAPHY

1. Bard, L. A. and Jarrett, W. H.: Intracranial complications of penetrating orbital injuries. Arch Ophth 71:332, 1964.

2. Goldberg, M. F. and Tessler, H. H.: Occult intraocular perforations from brow and lid lacerations. Arch Ophth 86:145, 1971.

3. Jones, L. T., Marquis, M. M., and Vincent, N. J.: Lacrimal function. Am J Ophth 73:658, 1972.

4. Silverman, J. P. and Obeare, M. F. : Delayed primary repair of totally avulsed upper and lower eyelids. Am J Ophth 70:230, 1970.

5. Rumelt, M. B. and Ernest, T. : Isolated blowout fracture of the medial orbital wall with medial rectus entrapment. Am J Ophth 73:451, 1972.

6. Werb, A. : Proceedings of the 2nd International Congress of Ophthalmology. Mosby, St. Louis, 1968.

7. Hale, L. M. : Povidone-Iodine in ophthalmic surgery. Ophth Surg 1:9, 1970.

8. Callahan, A. D. : Reconstructive surgery of the eyelids and ocular adnexa. Aesculapius, Birmingham, 1966.

9. Cutler, N. L. and Beard, C. : A method for partial and total upper lid reconstruction. Am J Ophth 39:1-7, 1955.

10. Bromberg, B. E. , Song, C. and Wladen, R. H. : Hydrotherapy of chemical burns. Plastic and Reconstructive Surg 35:85, 1965.

CHAPTER 10

STRESS INJURIES

Stress injuries are changes caused by abnormal barometric pressure, sudden variation in barometric pressure, and stress induced by vibration and acceleration.

An increase in atmospheric pressure produces cerebral symptoms because of higher partial pressure of gases in the blood and in the brain tissue and, in that way, causes visual disturbances. The toxic effect starts when the pressure is greater than two atmospheres.

A marked decrease in the barometric pressure results in anoxia. Functional changes in vision are more common than the organic effects. There may be loss in the visual acuity. Dilatation of pupils may be seen. The motor functions of the eyes may be impaired. Disturbances in accommodation and convergence also can be observed. Visual fields can be constricted and the stereoptic vision may be depressed.

Vasodilatation of the retinal vessels is among the early signs of anoxia caused by a subnormal barometric pressure. In the hypertensive subject, retinal hemorrhages may appear.

A sudden decrease in atmospheric pressure is the most important factor causing stress injuries. The disease so induced is called Caisson disease. Rapid release of air from the blood stream forms gas bubbles, causing micro emboli throughout the body. The general symptoms of rapid decompression are varied. Almost every organ can be affected.

Ocular symptoms are not too common; however, if they do occur, they are dramatic and serious. Subconjunctival, retinal, or choroidal hemorrhages may occur. Occasionally, the hemorrhage extravasates into the vitreous. Bubbles of gas can be seen in the vessels of the retina. The ophthalmoscopic appearance of central retinal occlusion is present (diffuse edema of the retina and a cherry-red macular spot). Paresis of the extraocular muscles or nystagmus is relatively common. The pupils may become irregular.

Functional visual phenomena such as defects in visual fields, flashlights, or complete amaurosis may occur, indicating embolic damage to the intracranial visual pathways and cortex.

Therapy is concentrated on prophylaxis. To prevent serious consequences it is important that the return from abnormal to normal barometric pressure is made gradually. If symptoms persist after return to normal atmospheric pressure, recompression must be undertaken at once and a slower decompression should be achieved.

GRAVITATIONAL AND VIBRATION STRESSES

Modern travel in high-speed airplanes and sudden acceleration or deceleration have introduced stress which may cause visual symptoms. Also, the human body is very sensitive to vibratory and gravitational stress such as are encountered during atmospheric or space flights or when a person is stationed at a piece of machinery for prolonged periods. Rapid vibration, about 40 cycles per second, reduces the visual acuity considerably. Changes in acceleration cause a drop in blood pressure, affecting the blood flow to the head and the eyes. Under these conditions, airplane pilots and astronauts report "greying" of vision. The more severe condition is the "black-out" or sudden and complete loss of vision which may be followed by unconsciousness.

Recovery from a "greying" or "black-out" is rapid. No residual abnormality of the visual system has been observed from repeated "black-outs." Therapy is not indicated in these cases and efforts should be concentrated on prophylaxis.

BIBLIOGRAPHY

1. Clark, B. and Graybiel, A.: Apparent rotation of a fixed target associated with linear acceleration in flight. Amer J Ophth 32: 549, 1949.

2. Duke-Elder, S.: System of Ophthalmology, Vol. XIV. Injuries. Henry Kimpton, London, and Mosby, St. Louis, 1972.

3. Graybiel, A.: Disorientation in pilots. Contact 5:412, 1945.

4. Symposium of the New Orleans Academy of Ophthalmology. Industrial and Traumatic Ophthalmology. Mosby, St. Louis, 1964.

5. Vinacke, W. E.: Illusions experienced by aircraft pilots while flying. J Aviation Med 18:308, 1947.

CHAPTER 11

RADIOLOGY OF OPHTHALMOLOGIC EMERGENCIES

Emergency x-ray in ophthalmology is usually limited to cases of trauma or inflammatory processes. The eyeball and the peribulbar tissue are involved in the case of a foreign body and the orbit itself requires x-ray examination when one suspects a fracture or an inflammatory or neoplastic process of the orbit.

Although the radiologic information is extremely important, it is helpful only if one realizes its limitations and recognizes the use to which it can be put.

To aid the emergency-room physician in solving ophthalmologic emergency problems, this chapter will present a short review of radiologic procedures, with special emphasis on cases of orbital fracture, location of intraocular foreign bodies, and some information concerning inflammatory and neoplastic processes extending to the bony orbit.

ANATOMY

Each orbit is roughly a four-sided pyramidal cavity located one on each side of the nasal cavity. The apex turns postero-medially and the base or "aditus" opens into the face. The orbit consists of seven bones and is divided into the roof, the lateral wall, the medial wall, and the floor.

The anatomy of the orbit is described briefly since its knowledge is essential to recognize pathologic conditions.

The roof separates the orbital cavity from the anterior fossa of the skull. It is formed anteriorly by the orbital part of the frontal bone and posteriorly by the lesser wing of the sphenoid bone. The trochlea of the superior oblique muscle is located antero-medially.

The lateral side of the roof turns downward to articulate with the greater wing of the sphenoid, these two forming the major part of the lateral wall. The anterior third of the lateral wall is formed by the zygomatic bone. The lateral wall is oblique, inclining in the latero-medial direction and proceeding from antero-lateral to postero-medial.

The medial wall is an almost vertical plane from the front to the back and is composed of the following structures: the frontal process of the maxilla, the lacrimal bone, the extremely weak lamina papyracea of the ethmoid and, posterior to the ethmoid, a small part of the body of the sphenoid.

The floor is formed mainly by the orbital plate of the maxilla, the orbital process of the zygomatic bone and, posteriorly, the orbital process of the palatine bone. The infraorbital groove is located in the middle of the floor leading into the infraorbital canal, transmitting the vessels and the infraorbital nerve (V-2) which exists through the infraorbital foramen immediately under the inferior rim of the orbit. The floor of the orbit consists of very thin bone, sometimes only 1 mm thick, and fractures easily.

The inferior orbital fissure is located between the floor and the lateral wall. The superior orbital fissure is near the apex, located between the lateral wall and the roof. Through this latter split, the III, IV, V-1, VI cranial nerves, sympathetic nerves, arteries and veins enter or leave the orbit.

The optic foramen, through which passes the optic nerve, is located at the apex of the orbit.

The base is bordered by the orbital rim which is formed by the frontal, zygomatic, and maxillary bones (Figs. 11-1, 11-2 and 11-3).

RADIOLOGIC TECHNIQUES

Radiographic examination of the orbits, as part of the skull, raises many difficult problems. Practically every single bone of the skeleton, except the skull, can be projected separately on the x-ray film and examined without any superimposition of other bony structures.

The skull is formed of 22 bones, and their close connection makes it technically impossible to obtain a separate projection of any one bone. Not only do the superimposed shadows of the adjacent bone structures cause difficulties in the interpretation of the x-ray film but also minimal changes in the positioning of the head at the time of exposure, markedly change the relationship of these shadows. Comparative anatomic studies have helped to work out methods to examine different structures.

The generally accepted procedures for radiographic examination of the orbits are the following:

The patient should be placed on the radiology table in a comfortable position without strain on the muscles and, when necessary, the body parts should be supported by pillows or sand bags. It is convenient to carry out the examination in the prone position. The head should be properly positioned. To maintain immobilization of the head, a clamp device, a weighted headband, or sand bags are used during the exposure. In order to avoid distortion of the picture, the film-target distance is approximately 36-40 inches. It is preferable to use a Potter-Bucky diaphragm to minimize scattered radiation. Usually, regular cassettes are equiped with intensifying screens.

It is impossible to give standard figures of exposure factors, that is, kilovolts (KV) and milliampere-seconds (MAS). Each make of x-ray equipment is different, therefore the exposure factors must be decided on the spot. These factors vary also according to the

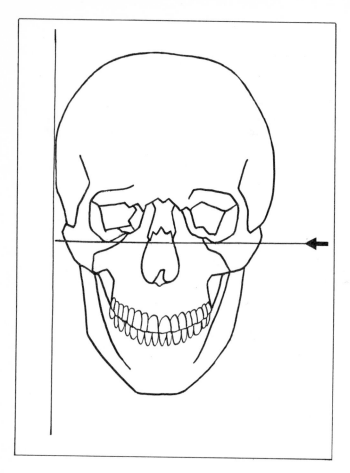

Fig. 11-1. Diagram of the normal skull. Direction of lateral x-rays.

thickness of the bone to be examined. For example, the bones of the young child are much thinner than those of the adult. Approximative values will be given for each individual view. Each x-ray technician, through his own experience with the equipment he uses, should know the precise amount of kilovolt and milliamper-seconds. Data given here is based on our experience.

Generally accepted routine methods are two exposures of postero-anterior positions of the orbits (the Caldwell view and Water's view), further on, one oblique of each side for comparison, and one lateral view of the affected side. If the above-mentioned techniques do not

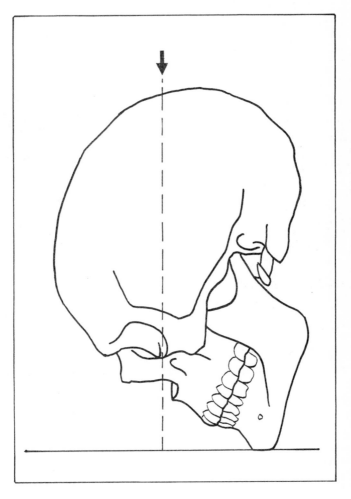

Fig. 11-2. Diagram of the normal skull. Direction of lateral postero-anterior x-rays.

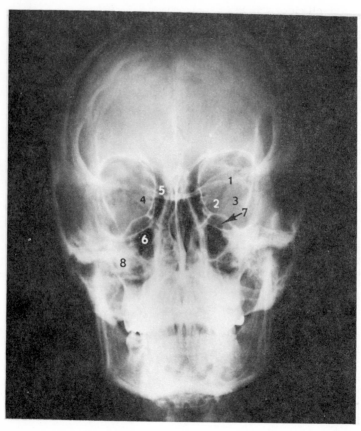

Fig. 11-3. Normal radiographic anatomic appearance of the skull.
An increased linear density, the sphenoid ridge, can be
seen inside the orbital rim. [1] The oblique slit is the
superior orbital fissure. [2] Lateral to this radiolucent
structure is the orbital surface of the sphenoidal greater
wing forming the lateral wall of the orbit. [3] Superomedi-
ally is the lesser wing. [4] Medially is the dark area
formed by the ethmoid cells. [5] Below the inferior rim
is the maxillary antrum. [6] A small hole projected on the
inferior rim is the intraorbital foramen. [7] The petrous
bone covers the lower third of the maxillary antrum. [8]

provide sufficient information, further variations of the positions are advisable; also, tomography may be used. The common positions are as follows:

1. Caldwell view. This modified and widely used form is a postero-anterior projection of the orbit. The patient is in the prone position and the head is placed in the straight (not tilted) face-down position so that the forehead and nose rest on the table. The cantho-meatal line is perpendicular to the plane of the film. (Canthus is the angle of the slit between the eyelids, inner or outer, and the meatus is the opening of the external auditory canal.)

The tube is tilted toward the feet so that the central ray is pointed to the glabella, forming a 15° angle with the cantho-meatal line. (Glabella is the area between the eyebrows.) (Figs. 11-4 and 11-5.)

The film-target distance is 40 inches; the approximate exposure factors, using cronex 4 film in par speed screen cassette, and Potter-Bucky diaphragm, are 75 to 78 KV, 80 to 84 MAS. During the exposure, respiration is suspended.

This position has the following advantages: a) The petrous ridges are projected downward and the orbital rim and roof are clearly visualized. b) The greater wing of the sphenoid (the major portion of the lateral wall) is easily detected. c) The orbital surface of the

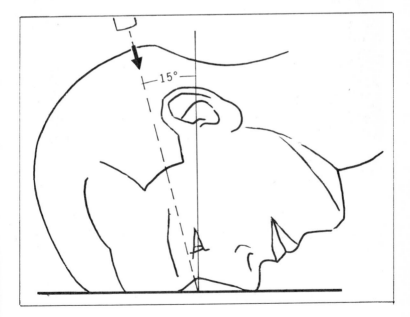

Fig. 11-4. Diagram showing direction of x-rays in the Caldwell view. The nose and forehead rest on the table, the cantho-meatal line is perpendicular to the plane of the film and the tube is tilted 15° caudally.

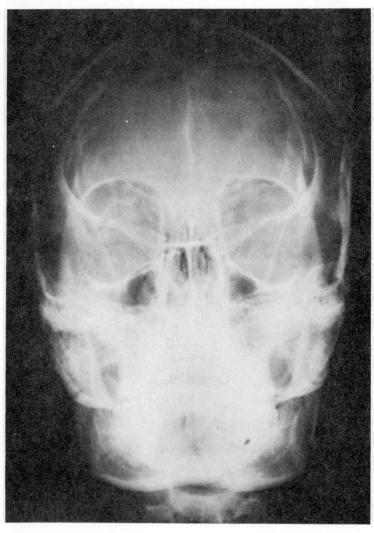

Fig. 11-5. Caldwell view. The orbital rim, the orbital roof, the greater wing and the lesser wing of the sphenoid, the superior orbital fissure, and the infraorbital foramen are visualized in this view.

lesser wing, as projected, can be seen close to the medial wall.
d) Between these two structures -- the greater and the lesser wings
of the sphenoid -- a relatively radiolucent slit of the superior orbital fissure is seen. e) The foramen rotundum is projected under the
inferior rim of the orbit (see Figs. 11-4 and 11-5).

2. <u>Water's view</u> is another postero-anterior position routinely used.
It allows additional visualization of the orbital and periorbital structures (Figs. 11-6 and 11-7). The patient is in the prone position so
that the sagittal plane is perpendicular to the plane of the table. The
head is extended so that the chin lies on the table above the lower
third of film cassette. In this position, the tip of the nose is raised
approximately 1 to 1-1/2 inches above the table. The main purpose
of the Water's view is to obtain a clear view of the maxillary antrum
from the superimposed petrous bones. If the head is extended too
far backward, the maxillary antrum is distorted. If the head is extended too far forward, the antrum is obscured by the projection of
the petrous bones. The best method is to adjust the cantho-meatal
line of the patient at an angle of 37° with the plane of the film. The
tube is centered above the vertex. The central rays are directed to
the midpoint of the film immediately below the nose on the anterior
nasal spine.

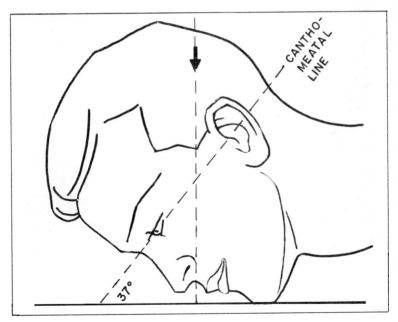

Fig. 11-6. Water's view. Diagram showing direction of x-rays. The
head is extended, the chin rests on the table. The nose
is raised approximately 1-1/2 inches. The cantho-
meatal line forms a 37° angle with the film. The central
beams exit below the nose.

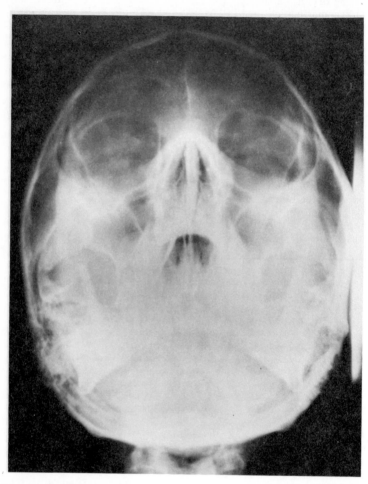

Fig. 11-7. Water's view. The inferior rim, the lateral wall of the
orbit, the superior orbital fissure, the zygomatic arch,
the frontal and ethmoidal sinuses are visualized. The
petrous bones are projected downward and the maxillary
antrum is clearly visualized.

The advantage of this view is that the petrous ridges are projected downward while the antral contours are complete and not deformed. Clear visualization of the maxillary antrum is of great help in revealing orbital pathology. The inferior orbital rim, the lateral wall, the zygomatic arch, and the frontal and ethmoidal sinuses are demonstrated on this view. The target-film distance is 40 inches, using cronex 4 film in par screen cassette. The exposure factors with the Potter-Bucky diaphragm are 80 to 82 KV, 80 MAS.

3. Oblique view is used to visualize the outer wall of the orbit and should be taken from both sides. The patient is positioned with the cheek, nose, and brow of the affected side resting on the table. The central rays enter through the occiput and exit through the center of the orbit. The advantage of this method is that it provides better visualization of the outer rim of the orbit (Fig. 11-8). Exposure factors are approximately 70 KV and 50 MAS.

The Rhese position of the orbit is useful to demonstrate the optic canal (Fig. 11-9). X-rays of this position should be taken from both sides separately for comparison. The patient is prone, his head adjusted so that the zygoma, nose, and chin on the respective side rest on the table.

Thus the head is rotated to the required side and the sagittal plane of the skull forms an angle of 53° with the plane of the film. The head is flexed somewhat until the acantho-meatal line is perpendicular to the plane of the film. (The acanthus is the area below the nose.)

The central rays follow the lateral canthus. The structures that are visualized are: the optic canal, appearing in the lateral inferior quadrant of the orbit, the ethmoid cells, the lesser wing of the sphenoid, and the superior orbital fissure. The target-film distance is 40 inches. Exposure factors are approximately 63 to 65 KV, and 50 MAS with Potter-Bucky diaphragm using cronex 4 film in par speed screen cassette.

If the patient is injured extensively and unable to assume the prone position, the film can be taken in the supine position. The head is turned toward the opposite side. The medio-sagittal plane of the head forms an angle of approximately 53° with the plane of the film. The central rays enter through the lower quadrant of the orbit to be examined. The contralateral orbit is examined in the same way, for comparison.

4. Lateral view is preferred to locate foreign bodies. The patient lies on his side, and the outer canthus of the respective orbit is placed on the film. The sagittal plane of the head is parallel with the plane of the film. The central rays are directed vertically through the canthus (Fig. 11-10). The exposure factors here, using cronex 4 film in par speed screen cassette without the Potter-Bucky diaphragm, are 50 to 55 KV and 10 MAS.

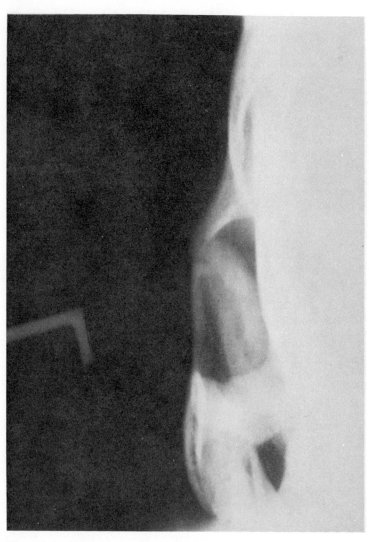

Fig. 11-8. Oblique view shows the external orbital rim and orbital border of the zygomatic bone.

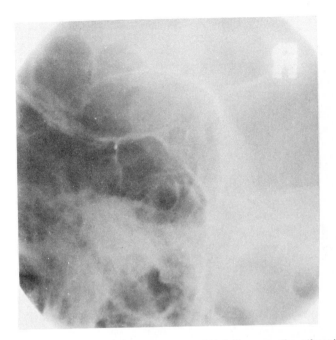

Fig. 11-9. Optic foramen, superior orbital fissure, the ethmoid
   cells, a portion of the medial wall.

5. If the above-mentioned views are not satisfactory for visualization of the orbital floor, a special method is offered by Fueger and
Milauskas. They found that the antero-lateral portion of the floor is
flat while the posterior one bulges. The patient is in nose-brow position, the cantho-meatal line is perpendicular to the plane of the
film, while the central rays angulate 30° caudally, much more than
in the previously described Caldwell technique. The central beams
come out one inch below the nasion. According to Fueger and
Milauskas, this offers better visualization of the posterior portion
of the orbital floor (Fig. 11-11). The antero-lateral part of the floor
is projected by an oblique view, when the patient's injured orbit is
adjusted to the cassette, approximately a 20° rotation of the head
toward the injured side. The glabello-meatal line is perpendicular
to the cassette and the central rays are angulated 35° so that they
come out near the tip of the nose (Fig. 11-12). These methods help
in the detection of a blow-out fracture of the orbital floor and have
the great advantage of revealing pathology of the orbits.

Occasionally, the patient is unable to sit or lie prone and we are
compelled to perform the examination in the supine position. In this
case, the head is immobilized and the tube is tilted caudally to eliminate the superimposition of the petrous bones and to obtain clearly
outlined orbits.

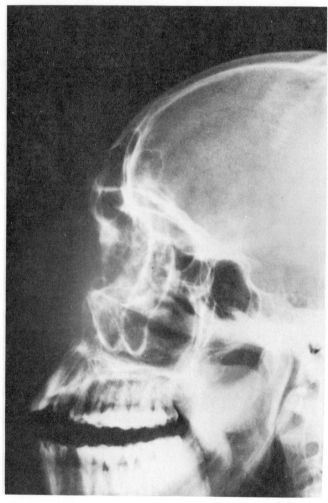

Fig. 11-10. Lateral view of the orbit.

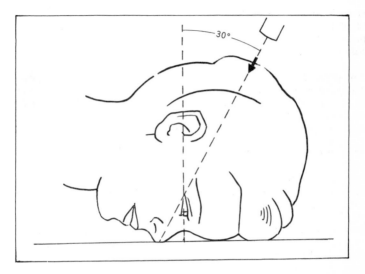

Fig. 11-11. Position suggested by Fueger-Milauskas. The nose and brow rest on the table. The tube is tilted caudally at an angle of 30° to the perpendicular.

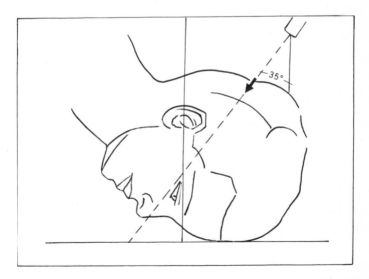

Fig. 11-12. The head is rotated toward the injured side. The rotation angle is approximately 20°. The glabello-meatal line is perpendicular to the cassette, the tube is tilted 35° caudally.

TOMOGRAPHIC TECHNIQUE

To eliminate the summation of image through the thickness of an anatomic structure, we use the technique of body-section radiography. By this method we can blur out the structures superimposing the desired area and clearly visualize a particular spot.

The principle is that during the exposure, the x-ray tube is moved in one direction above the area to be x-rayed and the film is moved in the opposite direction. The tube is adjusted so that the fulcrum is at the level of anatomic interest. This particular plane will be sharp against the blurred anatomic structures around it.

If the moving tube describes a greater arc, the plane of examination will be narrower. Linear tomography is relatively simple. If the tube angle is 30°, the movement is completed in 0.5 seconds (time and angles based on our polytome unit). If the angle is greater, more time is needed and the tomographic section will be thinner. To study the skeleton or structures that are not influenced by the patient's respiratory movements, a more sophisticated technique can be used that has the advantage of maximum blurring and thinner tomographic sections. Fortunately, the orbit lends itself to this procedure. To visualize pathologic changes in the orbit, particularly blow-out fractures which are hidden by overlying structures, different movements of the tube (circular, elliptical, hypocycloidal) are needed.

The best type of movement is hypocycloidal motion which describes a 48° arc, three eccentric circles, and gives a 1.3-mm thick plane. The time of exposure is six seconds. The advantage of this technique is that a sharper and thinner plane of focus is obtained.

The practical approach is to locate the tentative plane by linear tomography and, once oriented, to take a few sections with hypocycloidal motion. With linear tube movement, a 50° angle is used during 0.9 seconds, 75-80 KV and 75 MAS.

Hypocycloidal tomography requires a much longer exposure time -- 6 seconds, and 65 to 70 KV and 50 MAS.

COMPUTER-ASSISTED TOMOGRAPHY

A new diagnostic technique to examine the skull and its contents by computerized transverse axial tomography (ACTA scanner, EMI scanner) has been developed and introduced recently. Any part of the body can be scanned using this technique, but it is best suited to examine the skull.

Technically, the patient lies on an adjustable table and the head is placed within a rubber cap surrounded by a water-filled container. Increasing the amount of water, the cap is pressed firmly around the head and the air-gap is decreased to the minimum. The tomographic sections are taken parallel to Ried's baseline which is the line between the external auditory canal and the lower rim of the orbit. The patient's head is adjusted so that the line is perpendicular to the table top. Using a 0.8-cm thick slice, a few tomographic sections will provide complete visualization of the orbit. The collimated x-ray beam traverses the examined part and scans the horizontal planes. The x-ray tube detectors and collimeter are fixed to the same frame. The frame rolls through 180⁰ around the head in steps of 1⁰. The transmitted x-ray photons are received by a pair of sodium iodide crystals used as detectors instead of photographic film. The sodium iodide crystals are mounted on a photomultiplier installed opposite to the x-ray tube. The crystals emit visible light in proportion to the amount of photons reaching the detector and an electric signal is generated via a photomultiplier system. The x-ray source and detectors scan the head linearly, taking 160 readings in every step 1⁰ apart, through 180⁰, a total of 160 x 180. The data are stored on a magnetic disc or tape and analyzed on a viewing unit. Lesions are seen as a variation in tissue density differing from the surrounding normal. Tissue density enhancement can be achieved by using contrast media intravenously.

Computerized tomography has proved itself to be a revolutionary method in diagnostic radiology. It is very informative in globe injuries and retrobulbar hematoma. It is harmless and causes no discomfort to the patient. This brief description of the technique gives basic information and we hope that the unit, though very expensive, will be increasingly available.

FRACTURES OF THE ORBIT

The possible combination of fractures of the orbit are various and unpredictable. We will, however, try to describe them systematically, locating them according to the different anatomic structures of the orbit. The fractures are classified as follows:

1. Fracture of the middle facial structure
2. Fracture of the orbital rim
3. Blow-out fracture

The midfacial fractures were described by Réné Le Fort early in the twentieth century and his classification is in use today. Two of his groups involve the orbit. In the first group, Le Fort I, he described facial structures other than the orbit. In the second group, Le Fort II, a transverse fracture line runs forward through the nasal bones, the frontal process of the maxilla, the lacrimal bone, the orbital plate of the maxilla involving the infraorbital margin and turning downward on the anterior surface of the maxillary antrum. The fracture line passing backwards involves the posterior wall of the maxilla, the pterygomaxillary fissure, and continues through the pterygoid processes.

The third group, Le Fort III, includes the upper portion of the frontal process of the maxilla adjacent to the fronto-nasal and fronto-maxillary suture. It passes through the lacrimal bone and the ethmoidal plate, thus involving the medial wall of the orbit. The comminuting fracture lines usually do not extend to the optic foramen probably because the bone around it is quite dense. The line continues into the inferior orbital fissure and goes downward across the upper posterior aspect of the maxilla to the area of the spheno-palatine fossa and upward on the area of the zygomatico-sphenoid suture; thus, among other structures, the medial and lateral walls of the orbit are also involved. Fractures of the orbital rim usually result from a direct trauma.

Fracture of the roof and superior orbital rim can involve, in the latero-medial direction, the levator muscle, the supraorbital nerve, and the frontal sinus. It may be linear, extending into the frontal squamosa, or multiple, with possible extension to the deeper structures (dura, brain, etc.) (Figs. 11-13, 11-14, and 11-15).

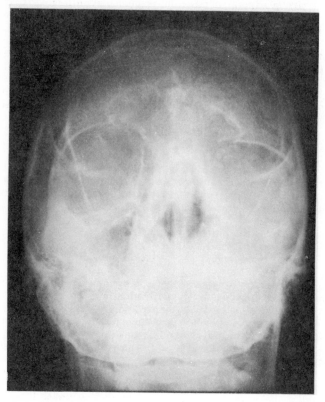

Fig. 11-13. The patient fell a distance of one flight. X-ray examination revealed a comminuted fracture of the left orbit, involving the upper rim, the roof, the frontal squamosa, and the outer wall. The soft tissue density over the maxillary and ethmoid area is increased. The entire picture suggests orbital fracture.

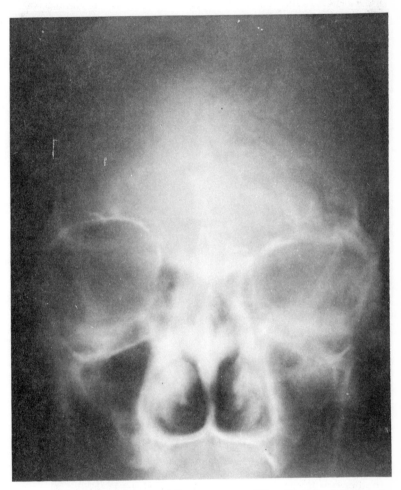

Fig. 11-14. Tomography of the same case (Fig. 11-13). Additional visualization of the fracture.

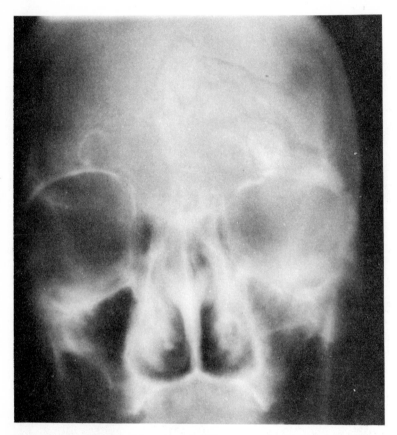

Fig. 11-15. Additional tomography (Fig. 11-14) shows the fracture
more clearly. Subsequent exploration confirmed the
x-ray diagnosis.

Fracture of the lateral wall and rim can involve the zygomatic frontal suture which is the weakest spot of the lateral wall. Fracture of
the lateral wall demands careful examination to detect additional
fractures of the zygomatic arch (Figs. 11-16 and 11-17).

Trauma of the zygomatic prominence will result in a fracture line
beyond the zygomatic maxillary sutural interface, continuing up-
wards to the antero-lateral surface of the maxillary antrum. The
fracture line continues through the infraorbital foramen backwards
on the infero-lateral portion of the orbital floor to the inferior orbital fissure.

A fracture which progresses to the postero-lateral wall of the
maxillary antrum results in a floating malar bone or "tripod" frac-

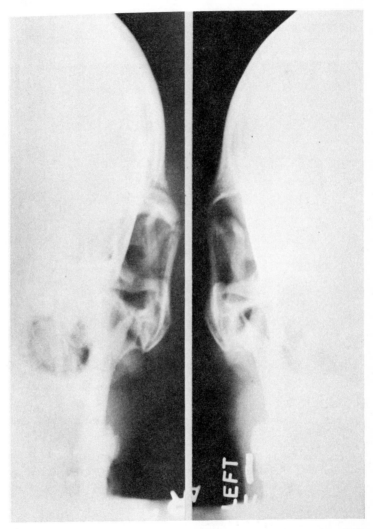

Figs. 11-16 and 11-17. Lateral wall fracture, as compared with the normal condition. Note the angulation of the zygomatic frontal suture area, with swelling of soft tissue.

ture. This demands immediate intervention because the infero-
lateral support of the eyeball is weakened by the mobile zygomatic
bone.

Fracture of the floor and inferior rim is due to direct trauma on the
continuation of the fracture lines from the medial or lateral wall.
The blow-out injury of the orbital floor will be described in greater
detail later (Fig. 11-18).

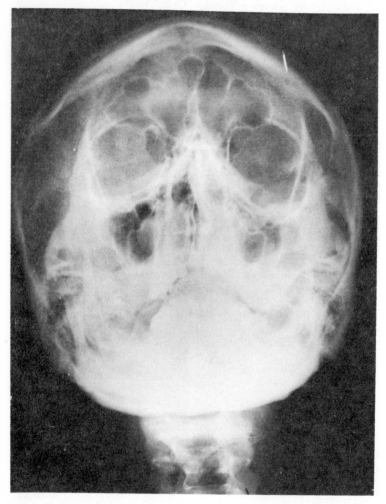

Fig. 11-18. Inferior orbital rim fracture indicated by interrupted
line. Note also increased density over the left half of
the nasal cavity.

Fracture of the nasal bone and frontal process of the maxilla can extend to the medial wall of the orbit. Fracture of the medial rim, as is blow-out fracture of the medial wall, is more common than recognized. Fracture of the medial wall can injure the nasolacrimal duct, the lacrimal sac, the medial canthal ligament, and the ethmoidal air cells. If it extends through the thin lamina papyracea to the cribriform plate, rhinorrhea occurs.

Blow-out fracture of the orbit differs from the previously described fractures. It can occur as part of a multiple facial fracture but it exists also as a specific syndrome as the only fracture of the facial skeleton. This occurs most frequently on the floor of the orbit, but recent reports in the literature call attention to blow-out fracture of the medial wall. The clinical symptoms manifesting themselves are quite minimal sometimes. The fracture should not be overlooked because it can cause irreversible damage to the oculomotor system of the injured side.

The pathogenesis of blow-out fractures is a suddenly increased intraorbital pressure due to a blow on the orbit by a convex object from the front. The power forces the intraorbital soft contents backwards without injuring the eyeball. The pressure is obviously transmitted equally to the walls and the fracture occurs at the weakest point of the orbit, such as the floor or the medial wall. Diagnosis of this kind of fracture of the floor is made more commonly than that of the medial wall, probably because of technical difficulties in visualizing precisely the structures of the medial wall. The mechanism of the medial wall blow-out fracture is similar to that of fracture of the floor. Epistaxis, subcutaneous emphysema, and retraction of the eyeball prevent adduction and usually call attention to the fracture of the extremely thin lamina papyracea. Pfeiffer assumes that the fracture occurs after the orbital contents compress the orbital floor. Le Fort supports the theory that the cause is the bone conduction through the rigid orbital rim to the thin floor. Regan supports the first theory calling this type "blow-out" or "hydraulic" fracture. With the sudden blow, the orbital contents press against the 1-mm thin floor.

Recently, several cases of concommitant blow-out fractures of the orbit and rupture of the eyeball were reported in the literature. This is an unusual complication. The pathomechanism of an injury such as this is not explained clearly. Dodick holds the same theory as Le Fort, adding that in certain cases the hitting force compresses the globe against the unyielding orbital wall, causing an increased intraocular pressure which leads to rupture.

The diagnosis should be based on the clinical and radiologic findings. The clinical symptoms of the blow-out fracture are discussed in further detail in Chapter 9. If a blow-out fracture is clinically suspected, the radiologist must confirm the diagnosis.

First, conventional positions such as Caldwell and Water's, and oblique views, and special positions to visualize the floor are taken.

If no pathology is seen, tomography might be helpful in the diagnosis (Fig. 11-19). If modern equipment is available, hypocycloidal tomography is a great help (Figs. 11-20 through 11-28).

An additional technique is the positive contrast orbitography. The procedure is as follows: 4 cc of 50% sodium diatrizoate (Hypaque) are mixed with 2 cc of xylocaine and hyaluronidase and injected along the inferior wall of the orbit, avoiding the muscle cone.

Immediately after the procedure, the patient is placed upright. If a blow-out fracture of the floor is present, the dye leaks into the maxillary antrum. Opinions differ as to the reliability of this method. If the needle is not inserted properly, that is, outside the muscle cone, the contrast medium will not penetrate through the fracture. Usually, the periorbital tissue of the injured side is severely swollen and it can be difficult not only to perform the procedure but also to interpret the results.

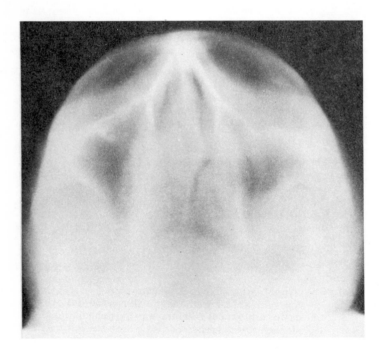

Fig. 11-19. The patient's left eye has been hit with a round object. Linear tomography reveals a blow-out fracture of the left orbital floor. Note and compare the uninterrupted orbital floor on the right.

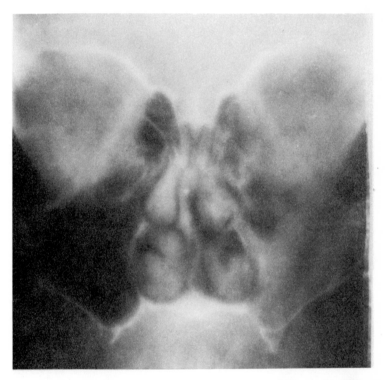

Fig. 11-20. Hypocycloidal tomogram, courtesy of Dr. A. Hornblass.
The patient had been hit by a fist in the left eye. Clinically, a blow-out fracture was suspected. Routine films
showed only increased density over the left maxillary
antrum. 14. 5-cm depth revealed only increased density.

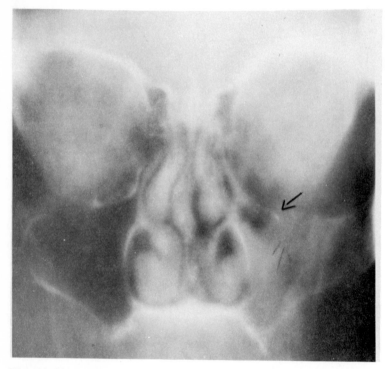

Fig. 11-21. Hypocycloidal tomogram, courtesy of Dr. A. Hornblass. The patient had been hit by a fist in the left eye. Clinically, a blow-out fracture was suspected. Routine films showed only increased density over the left maxillary antrum. 15-cm depth showed an interrupted line of the orbital floor (see arrow).

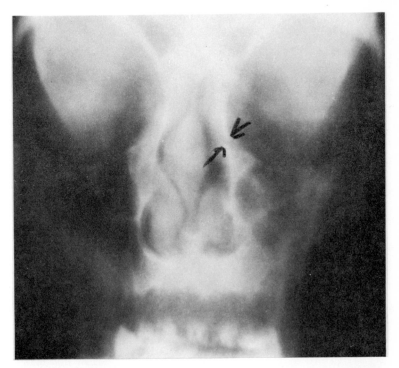

Fig. 11-22. Hypocycloidal tomogram, courtesy of Dr. A. Hornblass. The patient had been hit by a fist in the left eye. Clinically, a blow-out fracture was suspected. Routine films showed only increased density over the left maxillary antrum. 16.3-cm depth showed additional blow-out fracture of the medial wall (arrows).

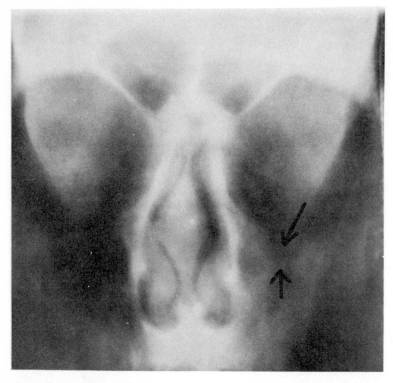

Fig. 11-23. Hypocycloidal tomogram, courtesy of Dr. A. Hornblass. The patient had been hit by a fist in the left eye. Clinically, a blow-out fracture was suspected. Routine films showed only increased density over the left maxillary antrum. 16.5-cm depth again shows clearly the blow-out fracture of the orbital floor.

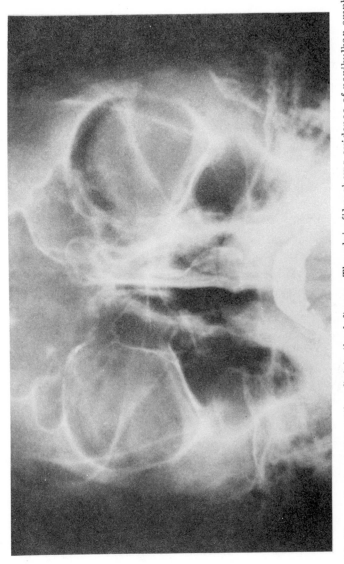

Fig. 11-24. The patient was hit with a fist in the left eye. The plain film shows evidence of peribulbar emphysema. There is an increased haziness in the area of the left ethmoid and nasal cavity. Note the intact maxillary antrum.

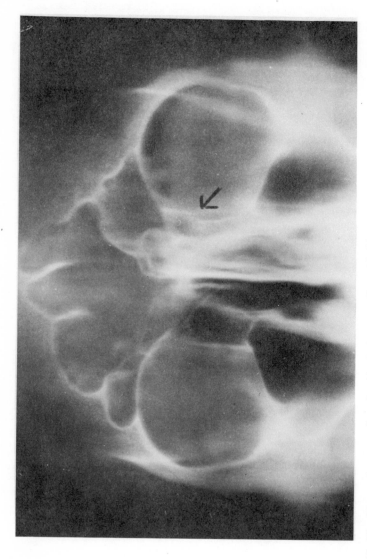

Fig. 11-25. Linear tomography of patient shown in Fig. 11-24 reveals a blow-out fracture of the medial wall.

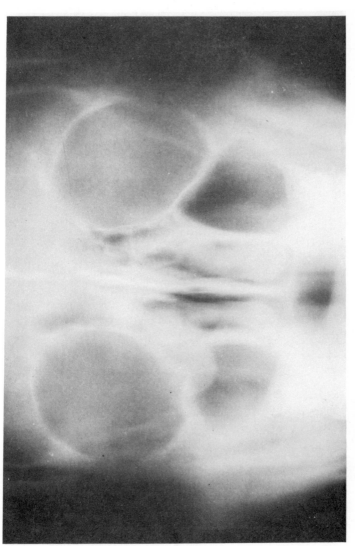

Fig. 11-26. Tomography of the orbit shows blow-out fracture of the anterior part of the right orbital floor. The round mass in the maxillary antrum is a protrusion of the peribulbar tissue (confirmed by surgery).

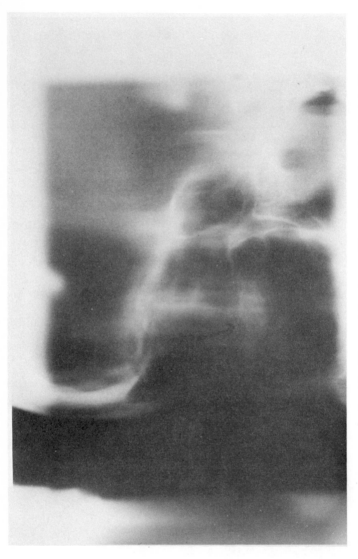

Fig. 11-27. Lateral tomogram of orbit. Blow-out fracture with soft tissue herniation into the maxillary antrum.

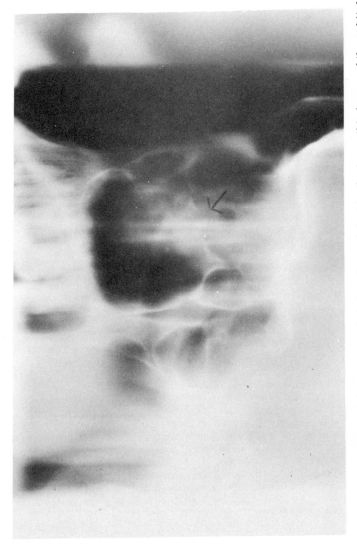

Fig. 11-28. Arrow on lateral tomogram points to a large defect in the inner third area of the orbital floor.

228/ Radiology of Ophthalmologic Emergencies

Recently, a rare type of fracture of the orbital floor, the so-called blow-in fracture, was described. Its etiology and clinical appearance is the same as that of the orbital blow-out fracture but, in this case, the floor is elevated.

FOREIGN BODIES

Locating a foreign body is a precise radiologic procedure which demands very accurate study by the radiologist. The presence of a radiopaque foreign body inside the globe is a potential danger.

The subject of retained intraocular foreign bodies such as iron or copper fragments is discussed in another section (Chapter 6). History of the accident is helpful in determining the chemical composition of the foreign body. Radiologically, however, there is no way to differentiate between iron, copper, stone, or lead-containing glass fragments. The experienced radiologist expects iron or copper to be more dense than a stone particle, but very often the foreign body is so small that its density does not indicate its chemical composition. In searching for an intraocular radiopaque foreign body, the first step is to obtain proper plain films of the orbits. To avoid "overdiagnostic interpretation," one should take two exposures on two different cassettes both in AP and lateral positions. Using this procedure, a false positive diagnosis caused by artifacts can be eliminated.

One should keep in mind that a phlebolyth, arterial calcification, or calcium deposit in the lens could appear occasionally on the plain film but careful radiologic and clinical examination of the patient will eliminate a false positive diagnosis.

Once it has been established that a foreign body is present in the orbital region, the next step is to determine its precise location and whether the particle is intra- or extraocular.

Approximately 30 different techniques are in use for the radiologic location of radiopaque foreign bodies. Most of these techniques require special and complicated accessory devices. The most commonly advised procedure is Sweet's method. The equipment consists of a metallic ball and a cone, each attached to a metallic rod, the two rods attached to another rod 15 mm apart. The patient lies on the affected side. The ball is placed 10 mm from the affected eyeball precisely in the center of the optical axis. A true lateral is taken; also, an oblique film is taken with the tube angled at 15-25° cranially. The location of the foreign body is then calculated from a specially prepared chart.

The Pfeiffer-Comberg method uses a contact lens placed on the cornea of the injured eye. The contact lens has four built-in opaque dots at 90° intervals indicating the limbus area (the corneoscleral junction). Postero-anterior and lateral exposures will show the location of the foreign body. By drawing circles approximately the size of the globe on both films, one can determine whether the foreign body is intra- or extraocular.

A slightly different technique was used successfully by C. W. Graham during World War II. A modified version of the Graham technique that was used successfully by the authors (Gombos and Hermann) with excellent results, in over 65 eye injuries, during the six-day Arab-Israeli War in 1967, will be described in detail. This technique does not require special apparatus and all the necessary accurate information can be obtained by usual x-ray technique.

The technique is as follows: under sterile conditions, using 5-0 or 6-0 silk, a metal ring is sutured around the corneoscleral junction of the anesthetized eye. (Only anesthetic eyedrops are used.) The diameter of the ring should be approximately 12 mm. X-ray exposures are taken while the patient fixates with the uninjured eye on a distant point. Two PA exposures are taken (Water's view) in gaze right and gaze left. Two lateral exposures are taken in upward gaze and in downward gaze (Figs. 11-29, 11-30, and 11-31). Frequently, one PA exposure and two lateral exposures, one in upward gaze and one in downward gaze, are as efficient as four exposures. If possible, the patient should be in the sitting position. It is very important to support the head to ensure immobility while the exposures are taken.

Interpretation is as follows: The diameter of the metal ring is known and is used to determine whether the films are magnified. If the anod-film distance is 30-35 inches, the magnification, if any, is probably not more than 0. 5 mm. The sagittal diameter of the eyeball is 24 mm. It is extremely important that the films be perfectly symmetrical so that the ring appears on the PA view as a perfect circle and on the lateral view as a vertical line, or almost so.

On the PA film, a circle of 12-mm radius is drawn around the geometric center of the metal ring. This circle approximates the size of the eyeball. On the lateral film, the 24-mm diameter eyeball is drawn from a point which is at a distance of 12 mm back from each end of the shadow of the metal ring on the film.

If the foreign body appears inside the circle in all films, it is most likely intraocular. Additional evidence is, if the foreign body moves with movement of the eye.

Whether the foreign body is anterior or posterior to the equator can be determined by studying the direction of movement of the foreign body. If it is identical with the direction of eye movement, the particle is anterior to the equator; if it is opposite, the foreign body is in the posterior half of the globe.

If the foreign body shows slight movements, it is probably either in Tenon's capsule or in episcleral tissue. If the foreign body does not move at all with movements of the eye, it is most likely extraocular.

The above described method has proved to be accurate in over 95% of cases.

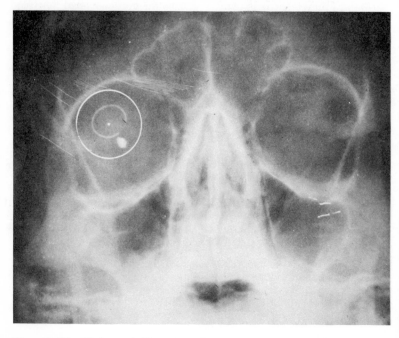

Fig. 11-29. History: A 25-year-old soldier was wounded by multiple
fragments from a hand grenade. His vision deteriorated
immediately after injury. Examination of the eyeball
revealed suspicious perforation of the sclera and cloudy
vitreous. The small circle indicates the metal ring sutured on the corneoscleral border. The outer circle,
drawn on the film later, indicates the outline of the eyeball. The increased metallic density between the two
circles is the foreign body. The small spot in the center
is an artifact.

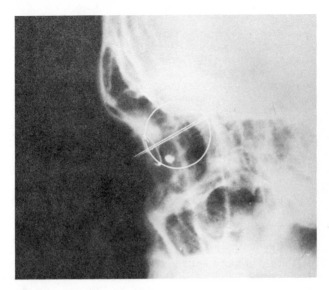

Fig. 11-30

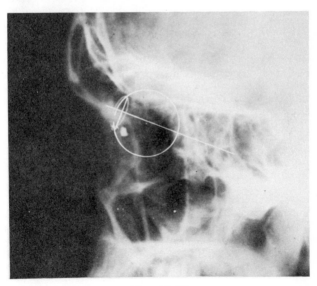

Fig. 11-31.

Figs. 11-30, 11-31. Lateral view in downward gaze and in upward gaze. The ring sutured on the corneoscleral boder indicates the level of the cornea. The drawn circle approximates the outline of the eyeball. The foreign body is intraocular and located anteriorly, since it follows the movements of the eye.

INFLAMMATIONS AND TUMORS

Inflammatory processes of the paranasal sinuses in the form of frontal, ethmoid, or maxillary sinusitis can occasionally involve an orbital wall, destroy it, and extend into the orbital content. The inflammation may sometimes occur spontaneously or it can be an unpleasant sequela of a previous surgical procedure. Usually, we can locate the inflammatory process and prevent its spread into the orbit. If the process is very active, it spreads rapidly through the bony orbit, menacing the orbital content. In such cases, early diagnosis and proper treatment will prevent progression of the inflammation.

In the early stage, the only x-ray finding is an increased density over the affected area due to the thickened mucosa or due to excessive secretion into the accessory nasal cavity.

The minimal atrophy manifests itself early as irregular, moth-eaten appearance of the bones around the orbit. This appearance may be an indication of destruction of the floor due to an extension of a maxillary antral process into the orbit, or destruction of the lamina papyracea due to extension of the process from the ethmoid air cells into the orbit. Also, it may be due to an inflammatory or neoplastic process extending from the frontal sinus through the adjacent superomedial wall of the orbit. These radiologic signs are characteristic also of an inflammatory or neoplastic process originating in the accessory nasal cavity and affecting the orbit.

Because the superimposed soft tissue shadow can obscure the early bone changes, tomography of the orbit is advisable as it will reveal the bone destruction. The use of tomography and early diagnosis is important because surgical exploration can prevent damage and the subsequent irreversible changes in the affected eye.

Another, fortunately rare, pathologic change is malignant neoplasm of the paranasal sinuses. Tumors extending to the orbit usually originate in the maxillary antrum or in the ethmoid cells. Primary carcinoma is the most common disease but sarcomas also occur.

Tumors involving the orbit are the following:
a) Tumors of the nasal cavity at the level of the inferior surface of the superior turbinate.
b) Tumors of the maxillary antrum involving the entire mucosal lining (endosinus) that originate above the level of the middle turbinate (suprastructure) and may spread into the orbital cavity causing proptosis due to the retrobulbar tumorous mass. The radiologic pictures in each of these two types show a huge soft tissue mass with destruction of the orbital floor (Figs. 11-32 and 11-33).
c) Ethmoid sinus tumor spreading through the medial orbital wall into the orbit.
d) Frontal sinus tumor spreading through the upper medial orbital wall into the orbit.

The most common factor in all these neoplasms is the prominent swelling of soft tissue and destruction of the corresponding bony structure. In the acute stage, it is almost impossible to differentiate radiologically between bone destruction due to malignant disease and that due to an inflammatory process. Thus, surgical exploration is inevitable.

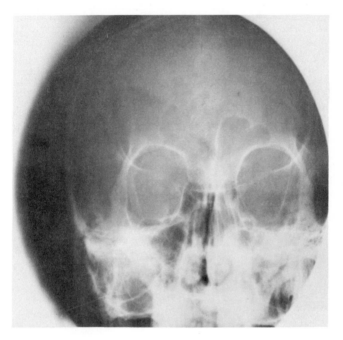

Fig. 11-32. Caldwell view

Figs. 11-32, Caldwell view, and 11-33, Water's view. A 50-year-old male was admitted to the emergency room six days after a tooth extraction. Clinical findings included a markedly swollen left face and periorbital tissue, as well as marked exophthalmus. Radiologic picture shows increased density over the left maxilla, the ethmoid, and the left part of the nasal cavity. The inferior orbital rim is indistinct. However, based on this examination, no evidence of bony destruction was detected.

The clinical and radiologic findings were suspicious of an inflammatory, eventually of a malignant, process and demanded surgical exploration which subsequently confirmed the diagnosis of carcinoma of the antrum extending into the orbit.

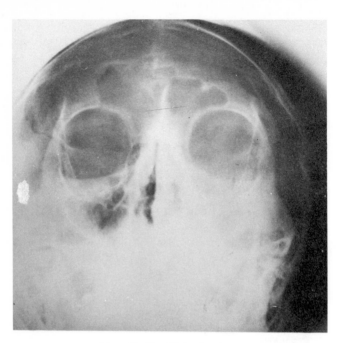

Fig. 11-33. Water's view

BIBLIOGRAPHY

1. Athanasiu, M. : Direct roentgen location on the sclera-surface of marginal foreign bodies with the aid of special grids. Ophthalmologica Additamentum 158:325, 1969.

2. Beisner, D. H. : Orbital radiography. Surv Ophth 13:187, 1968-69.

3. Bronson, N. R. : Nonmagnetic foreign body localization and extraction. Am J Ophth 58:133, 1969.

4. Converse, J. M. and Byron, S. : Naso-orbital fractures. Trans Am Acad Ophth & Otolaryng 67:622, 1963.

5. Diwan, R. , Sen, D. K. and Sood, G. C. : Rat bite orbital cellulitis. Brit J Ophth 54:211, 1970.

6. Dodick, J. M. , Littleton, J. T. and Sod, L. M. : Concomitant medial wall fracture and blow-out fracture of the orbit. Arch Ophth 85:273, 1971.

7. Dodick, J. M. , Galin, M. A. and Kwitko, M. L. : Concomitant blow-out fracture of the orbit and rupture of the globe. Arch Ophth 84:707, 1970.

8. Dodick, J. M. , Berrett, A. and Galin, M. A. : Hypocycloidal tomography and orbital blow-out fracture. Am J Ophth 68:483, 1969.

9. Dodick, J. M. , Galin, M. A. and Berrett, A. : Radiographic techniques in the diagnosis of blow-out fracture of the orbit. Ann Ottalmol Clin Ocul 95:577, 1969.

10. Dodick, J. M. , Galin, M. A. and Berrett, A. : Radiographic evaluation of orbital blow-out fracture. Can J Ophthal 4:370, 1969.

11. Dodick, J. M. , Galin, M. A. and Kwitko, M. : Medial wall fracture of the orbit. Can J Ophth 4:377, 1969.

12. Dodick, J. M. , Berrett, A. and Galin, M. A. : Hypocycloidal tomography of the orbit. Surgical Forum 19:484, 1968.

13. Etter, L. E. et al. : Atlas of Roentgen Anatomy of the Skull. C C Thomas, Springfield, Ill. , 1970.

14. Ferguson, E. D. : Deep, wooden foreign bodies of the orbit. Trans Am Acad Ophth & Otolaryng 74:778, 1970.

15. Fischbein, F. I. and Lesko, W. S. : Blow-out fracture of the medial orbital wall. Arch Ophth 81:162, 1969.

16. Fueger, G. F. , Milauskas, A. T. and Britton, W. : The roentgenologic evaluation of orbital blow-out injuries. Am J Roentgenol 97:614, 1966.

17. Fletcher, G. H. and Jing, Bao-Shan: The Head and Neck. Year Book Medical Publishers, Chicago, 1968.

18. Gahagan, L. O. : Roentgenologic examination of the orbit. EENT Monthly 41:915, 1962.

19. Gawler, J. et al. : Computer assisted tomography in orbital disease. Brit J Ophth 58:571, 1974.

20. Gould, H. R. and Titus, C. O. : Internal orbital fractures: the value of laminagraphy in diagnosis. Am J Roentgenol 97:618, 1966.

21. Gregory, E. M. : An unusual case of blow-out fracture of the orbit. Med J Aust 2:802, 1969.

22. Havener, W. H. and Gloeckner, S. L. : Atlas of Diagnostic Techniques and Treatment of Intraocular Foreign Bodies. Mosby, St. Louis, 1969.

23. Hounsfield, G. N. : Computerized transverse axial scanning (tomography): Part I. Description of system. Brit J Radiol 46: 1016, 1973.

24. Howard, G. M. : The orbit. Arch Ophth 82:851, 1969.

25. Industrial and Traumatic Ophthalmology. Symposium of the New Orleans Academy of Ophthalmology. Mosby, St. Louis, 1964.

26. Lampert, L. V. , Zelch, J. V. and Cohen, D. N. : Computed tomography of the orbits. Radiology 113:351, 1974.

27. Lerman, S. : Blow-out fracture of the orbit. Diagnosis and treatment. Brit J Ophth 54:90, 1970.

28. Littleton, J. T. and Witner, F. S. : Linear laminagraphy. Am J Roentgenol 95:981, 1965.

29. Lombardi, G. and Passerini, A. : The orbit and contrast media. Arch Ophth 78:306, 1967.

30. Merrell, R. A. and Yanagisawa, E. : Radiographic anatomy of the paranasal sinuses. Arch Otolaryng 87:184, 1968.

31. Merrill, V. : Atlas of Roentgenolgraphic Positions, vol. 2, 3rd ed. , Mosby, St. Louis, 1967.

32. Milauskas, A. T. , Fueger, G. F. and Schulze, R. R. : Clinical experiences with orbitography in the diagnosis of orbital floor fractures. Trans Am Acad Ophth & Otolaryng 70:25, 1966.

33. Momose, K. J. et al. : The use of computed tomography in ophthalmology. Radiology 115:361, 1975.

34. Patterson, C. N. : Siliconized dacron implants in septal and orbital surgery. Arch Otolaryng 89:71, 1969.

35. Pfeiffer, R. L. : Localization of intraocular foreign bodies by means of the contact lens. Arch Ophth 32:261, 1944.

36. Pfeiffer, R. L. : Localization of intraocular foreign bodies with the contact lens. Am J Roentgenol 44:558, 1940.

37. Potter, G. D. and Trokel, S. : Tomography of the optic canal. Am J Roentgenol 106:530, 1969.

38. Roberts, W. E. : The roentgenographic demonstration of glass fragments in the eye. Am J Roentgenol 66:44, 1951.

39. Romanes, G. J. : Cunningham's Textbook of Anatomy, 10th ed. Oxford University Press, London, 1964.

40. Rowe, N. L. and Killey, H. C. : Fractures of the Facial Skeleton, 2nd ed. Williams and Wilkins, Baltimore, 1968.

41. Runyan, T. E. and Levri, E. A. : Vitreous analysis in eyes containing copper and iron intraocular foreign bodies. Am J Ophth 69:1053, 1970.

42. Schultze, R. C. : Supraorbital and glabellar fractures. Plastic and Reconstructive Surgery 45:227, 1970.

43. Seymour, E. Q. and Bane, D. B. : A comparison of the accuracy of the Comberg and Sweet techniques of orbital foreign body localization. Radiol 96:75, 1970.

44. Shanks, S. C. and Kerley, P. : Textbook of X-ray Diagnosis, 3rd ed. , vol. 1. Saunders, Philadelphia, 1957.

45. Smith, B. and Regan, W. F. : Blow-out fracture of the orbit. Am J Ophth 44:733, 1957.

46. Stallard, H. G. : War surgery of the eye. An analysis of 102 cases of intraocular foreign bodies. Brit J Ophth 28:105, 1944.

47. Sweet, W. M. : Improved apparatus for localizing foreign bodies in the eyeball by the roentgen rays. Trans Am Ophth Soc 12: 320, 1909.

48. Symposium on Radiology of the Orbit. Radiol Clinics of N Am 10:No. 1, April, 1972, W. N. Hanafee, ed.

49. Trokel, S. L. and Potter, G. D. : Radiographic Diagnosis of fracture of the medial wall of the orbit. Am J Ophth 67:772, 1969.

50. Vinik, M. and Gargano, F. P. : Orbital fractures. Am J Roentgenol 97:607, 1966.

51. Wright, J. W. and Taylor, C. C. : A valuable aid to diagnosis of ear disease: Hypocycloidal polytomography. J Indiana State Med 63:29, 1970.

CHAPTER 12

NEURO-OPHTHALMOLOGIC EMERGENCIES

INTRODUCTION

Neuro-ophthalmology is the discipline of ophthalmology which is concerned with the ocular manifestations of neurologic disease. Many neurologic entities have significant eye signs and can be diagnosed on the basis of those eye signs. It has been stated that approximately 38% of all nerve fibers in the central nervous system are concerned with visual function. In addition to the direct pathways with which the above statement is concerned, the visual impulse from the retinal receptor to the occipital pole is influenced by other regions of the brain. The concept of vision includes visual attention and recognition, the registration of memory, as well as cortical influences on ocular movement. The lengthy and circuitous course of the visual pathways in the brain also brings them in close proximity with many important cerebral structures.

Dysfunction of the cerebral hemispheres, optic chiasm, diencephalon, midbrain, pons and medulla can produce defects in visual or oculomotor function. Diseases of the cerebral hemispheres and optic chiasm produce characteristic visual field abnormalities which help in localization. Visual field defects are accurate indicators of the localization of intracranial lesions. Almost always, a homonymous field defect is a reflection of disease in the opposite cerebral hemisphere in its posterior two-thirds. The "classical" indicators of lesions on one side of the brain or the other can be misleading. Usually, a left Babinski sign is found with a right cerebral lesion, but in some cases, a left Babinski sign can occur in a left cerebral lesion. This is rarely the finding with visual field defects. A left homonymous hemianopia is a reliable indicator of a right cerebral lesion and its visual radiation, that portion of the visual pathway between the lateral geniculate body and the occipital lobe with its ramifications in the temporal and parietal subcortical regions.

Increased intracranial pressure is reflected in the ophthalmoscopic finding of papilledema. Moreover, the presence of sudden loss of vision associated with a papillitis is visible on funduscopic examination. A retrobulbar neuritis can be diagnosed by the presence of a marked central scotoma. The evaluation of the extraocular and intraocular muscles is an important aspect of the diagnosis of brainstem dysfunction.

Eight of the twelve cranial nerves are concerned with the eye. Cranial nerve I consists of the olfactory nerve and tract. Intracranial disease impairing function of the olfactory tract commonly produces findings related to optic nerve or optic chiasm dysfunction. The second cranial nerve, or the optic nerve, is concerned with direct transmission of the visual impulse from the external environment to the brain. The afferent portion of the light reflex is also transmitted via the optic nerve. Cranial nerves III, IV, and VI participate in regulation of ocular motility. A portion of the 8th cranial nerve, the vestibular nerve, plays an important role in influencing ocular motility. The first division of the fifth cranial nerve is the nerve transmitting sensation from the cornea. Portions of the maxillary division of the trigeminal nerve also play a significant role in visual function. The facial or 7th cranial nerve mediates eye closure and, thus, protection of the eye.

NEURO-OPHTHALMOLOGIC EXAMINATION

The neuro-ophthalmologic examination includes elements of both the ophthalmologic as well as the neurologic examinations. Since both focal and diffuse disease of the nervous system can affect the visual system, the techniques of the neurologic examination are important in arriving at a neuro-ophthalmologic diagnosis. However, the use of the biomicroscope, indirect ophthalmoscopy, as well as visual field techniques, are also important in arriving at a diagnosis.

As in all fields of medicine, the history is perhaps the most important part of the examination. The patient may complain of transient visual loss in either one or both eyes. Transient loss of vision in one eye, amaurosis fugax, is an important symptom of carotid artery disease on the ipsilateral side. Obscurations are also phenomena of visual loss in one eye but usually occur with papilledema, particularly when it has been chronic. Transient visual loss of both eyes can indicate migraine, or the hemianopic attacks of ischemia in the vertebrobasilar arterial system. The intolerance of bright light or photophobia can occur in the absence of ocular disease. It occurs with concussion, meningitis, and subarachnoid hemorrhage. Moreover, it has also been noted during the recovery phase of infarctions involving the visual pathways supplied by the middle cerebral artery. Another important historical point of information is the presence of visual hallucinations. Unformed visual hallucinatory experiences indicate lesions of the occipital or parieto-occipital lobes. Formed visual hallucinations indicate temporal lobe disease. However, visual hallucinations can be confused with entoptic phenomena, such as "spots" in front of the eyes, or "lightning flashes" in the periphery of the visual field. This may be related to stimulation of the retina by vitreo-retinal traction.

The symptom of diplopia is alarming. Patients complain of blurred vision when indeed they are referring to double vision. The presence of horizontal diplopia usually indicates unilateral or bilateral sixth nerve disease. The diplopia is usually more prominent for distance than for near. Involvement of the third or fourth cranial nerves usually produces vertical diplopia. Transient diplopia may indicate vertebrobasilar disease. Permanent diplopia can occur with lesions in the orbit, neural pathways or brain-stem nuclei. Monocular diplopia can be of local ocular origin such as keratoconus, cataract, macular lesions, or astigmatic refractive errors.

Patients with neuro-ophthalmologic disease also complain of reading problems. It is important to differentiate whether the reading difficulty occurs at the beginning of the line or at the end of the line. Metamorphopsia refers to distortion of vision. Images may appear smaller, larger, tilted, or closer or farther in the environment. Constant metamorphopsia indicates lesions of the retina, whereas the intermittent nature of metamorphopsia is a reflection of intracranial disease, usually involving the geniculocalcarine pathways. Oscillopsia is the illusory movement of the environment and is a complaint of patients with brainstem dysfunction. Most patients with oscillopsia also demonstrate nystagmus in the primary position.

Frequent changes in refraction may be the initial indication of a chiasmal lesion. Patients with disorders in the region of the optic chiasm may also present with difficulty in recognizing familiar faces, the phenomenon of prosopagnosia. However, this may also be a complaint of patients with parietal lobe disease.

Initially, it is important to obtain an idea of the patient's visual acuity. It should be remembered that patients with neurologic disease, particularly those with bilateral cerebral dysfunction, may deny their inability to see, which is accompanied by a confabulation of the images of the environment. If a patient can read ordinary newspaper print, the visual acuity is approximately 20/50. If headlines can be read, the acuity is 20/200. If the patient requires a refractive correction, an estimate of the optimum visual acuity can be obtained by using a "pin-hole." The vision should be recorded even if the patient is only able to count fingers, perceive hand motion or light. If the patient makes no attempt to read whatsoever, consideration must be given to the presence of dyslexia which may indicate the presence of parietal lobe disease.

Examination of the visual fields is occasionally difficult in patients suffering from neurologic disease, since the neurologic dysfunction not uncommonly involves the ability to concentrate. Thus, formal perimetric or tangent screen examinations may be inaccurate. Reliance must then be placed upon methods involving techniques of confrontation to elicit abnormalities. Simultaneous targets are presented in the superior and inferior nasal and temporal quadrants to either eye while the other is occluded. There is a spectrum of defects which can be elicited, in which color targets are most sensitive. Perception of motion and form may be preserved when the perception of color targets has become impaired because of a visual field defect. Since the evaluation of the patient with neuro-ophthalmologic disease may take place in an emergency room situation, methods which can produce a rapid and adequate description of the patient's vision with simple apparatus are important. However, conventional perimetry gives a more accurate outline of the visual field defect. The clinical evaluation of the visual fields includes examination for hemispatial agnosia wherein the patient ignores one-half of the visual field. Patients may voluntarily mention the fact that they perceive only part of the examiner's face. A Snellen eye chart or a page of words can also be used. Finger movement, counting fingers, visualization of matches, and the response to threatening gestures can also be used as instruments for evaluation of the visual field. Pseudoisochromatic plates are also helpful in the evaluation of the visual field in the presence of a gross visual field defect. Patients ignore the digit on the side of the defective visual field. Thus, a patient with a left homonymous defect will report 74 as 4, 12 as 2, or, in the case of number 8, it will be reported as 3. If the patient cannot speak, ask him to trace what he sees. Failure to report both digits correctly when the test is performed accurately in the other eye indicates a central scotoma or other central visual field defect. Approximately 30 to 40% of patients with homonymous defects will make errors using this method and therefore it cannot be relied upon to exclude lesions of the visual pathways.

The pupillary reactions should be evaluated as to their response both directly and consensually. The swinging flashlight sign or Marcus-Gunn pupillary phenomenon should be evaluated for the presence of optic nerve or retinal dysfunction. The responses of the pupil to convergence and accommodation is also essential. Presence of ptosis associated with a large pupil indicates third nerve dysfunction and ptosis with a small pupil would indicate a Horner's syndrome. With a Horner's syndrome, the lower lid of the involved side is also somewhat higher than on the normal side. The lower lid margin thus covers a larger segment of the limbus of the involved eye. The pupil in a patient suffering from angle-closure glaucoma will be large and occasionally asymmetric. In a patient suffering from a severe headache, which may mimic increased intracranial pressure, the pupil is usually miotic.

Examination of ocular movements includes the all important corneal reflex. Lesions within the cavernous sinus including inflammation, aneurysms and metastatic tumors will impair function of the ophthalmic division of the 5th cranial nerve. Cerebellopontine angle tumors will also impair function of the ophthalmic nerve. Herpes simplex and herpes zoster involvement of the cornea will produce decreased corneal sensation. A bilateral decrease of corneal sensation is usually not significant. The eyelids should be observed for the size and width of the palpebral fissures as well as the spontaneity of opening and closing movements. The tone of the eyelids should also be noted. Patients in the state of early coma resist passive eye opening. A doughy tone of the eyelids, when they are raised and observed to fall slowly back into place, indicates a deeper state of coma.

The primary position of the eyes should be noted as well as the ability to converge. Gross ocular malalignment and apraxia of ocular movement should be noted. Conjugate ocular movements should be evaluated on demand (both horizontally and vertically) on pursuit and, on command, to look at specific objects or targets. Oculocephalic maneuvers in the horizontal and vertical position should be performed and the presence of Bells phenomenon noted. The presence of nystagmus, both spontaneous and with movement, should be evaluated. Investigation for positional nystagmus, vestibular nystagmus, as well as impairment of optokinetic nystagmus is essential. Applanation tonometry is part of the neuro-ophthalmologic evaluation.

Auscultation and palpation of the vessels of the neck should be performed. Auscultation over the orbits, neck, and cranium can reveal evidence of cerebrovascular disease. Bruits over the ipsilateral carotid artery occur in approximately 60 to 70% and over the contralateral artery in about 10% of patients with carotid occlusive disease. Bruits over the orbits can be found with both a carotid-cavernous fistula and a vascular malformation, intracranially.

The performance of ophthalmodynamometry is considered by some authorities to be useful in the evaluation of carotid vascular disease. However, it should be remembered that an asymmetry in the findings of ophthalmodynamometry usually indicates sufficient narrowing of the lumen of the carotid artery to produce an approximate 60 to 80% compromise in the lumen. A normal ophthalmodynamometric finding by no means excludes the presence of carotid artery disease.

A funduscopic and retinal examination can reveal evidence of retinitis pigmentosa, cerebromacular degeneration, and the neurophakomatoses. Moreover, yellow or white refractile bodies can be noted in the lumen of retinal arterioles following embolization from carotid artery thrombi. The optic discs should be evaluated for the presence of papilledema, medullated nerve fibers, drusen, or other congenital defects. Optic atrophy can occur with either primary retinal or with primary neurologic disease. It may also follow an optic neuritis or papilledema.

CLASSIFICATION OF DISEASE

The importance of anatomically localizing the region of neurologic dysfunction is based upon the fact that management and prognosis depend upon the specific anatomic region involved.

Dysfunction of the cerebrum may be recognized by the presence of convulsions or paroxysmal disturbances of cerebral function. Mental and behavioral changes of the organic type are also seen in cerebral disease. Aphasia, homonymous visual field defects, and hemiplegia are other neurologic findings in patients with disease of the cerebral hemispheres.

Dysfunction of the basal ganglia is revealed in the presence of dyskinesias, such as tremor, choreiform movements, athetosis and hemiballismus. Alterations in tone, posture, and movement are also found with basal ganglia disease.

Dysfunction of the cerebellum is manifested by unsteadiness in motor performance, such as alterations in gait, dysdiadokokinesis, asynergia, ataxia, unchecked rebound, as well as past-pointing.

Involvement of the brainstem, which includes the midbrain, pons, and medulla, produces nystagmus, both horizontal and vertical.

Bilateral pupillary paralysis, defects in articulation, phonation, vocalization, swallowing, and tongue movements are also seen with brainstem disease. Crossed syndromes, which include paralysis of eye movements, face, or tongue on one side, with sensory defects on the opposite side of the body, are also seen in brainstem disease.

An etiologic classification of neuro-ophthalmologic disease should consider the presence of (a) vascular, (b) neoplastic, (c) toxic-metabolic, (d) infectious, (e) traumatic, (f) genetic and de-generative, (g) congenital and developmental, (h) osseous and muscular, (i) idiopathic, and (j) psychogenic disorders.

The determination of the anatomic site as well as the possible etiologic causes will influence the type of examination which should be performed. A complete blood count, urinalysis, chest x-ray, and lumbar puncture should be performed routinely. Studies of the cerebrospinal fluid, including cytology and serology, total cell count with differential, total protein and globulin values, are important. Other examinations which may have to be performed include skull series, electroencephalography, brain scan, echoencephalography, computerized transaxial tomography, angiography, and pneumoencephalography (Table 1).

TABLE 1

TESTS FOR NEURO-OPHTHALMOLOGIC DISEASE

1. X-rays of the skull
2. Electroencephalography
3. Echoencephalography
4. Radioactive isotope encephalography (brain scan)
5. Computerized transaxial tomography
6. Angiography
7. Pneumoencephalography
8. Ventriculography
9. Cerebrospinal fluid studies (lumbar puncture)
   A. Appearance of cerebrospinal fluid
   B. Pressure
   C. Total protein; gamma globulin
   D. Cell count
   E. Cytology
   F. Serology
   G. Culture and sensitivity; acid fast stain
   H. India ink preparation
10. X-rays of spine
11. Myelography

An ocular emergency may be defined as any situation which is either a threat to vision, has caused loss of vision, or has produced severe eye pain or deformity. The definition of a neuro-ophthalmologic emergency can be extended to include the ocular emergency plus the threat, or actual occurrence, of permanent dysfunction of the brain and thus the life of the individual. Neuro-ophthalmologic emergencies can usually be diagnosed on the basis of disordered functioning of the visual or oculomotor systems. Emergencies such as occlusion of the central retinal artery usually require the institution of immediate therapy. The evaluation of a patient with possible temporal arteritis requires both an accurate history, test for specific neuro-ophthalmologic abnormalities, as well as confirmation of its existence by an abnormal E. S. R. The differentiation of papilledema from optic neuritis should be performed with great care in order to preclude the performance of several unnecessary and discomforting examinations. Most neuro-ophthalmologic emergencies require accurate and repeated evaluation with the institution of a specific course of action once a diagnosis is established.

The eye and its adnexae are subject to injury from head trauma. Evaluation and treatment of "blow-out" fractures of the floor of the orbit will be discussed in another chapter.

DIRECT INJURY

The "black eye" is a hematoma in the eyelids and is evidence of direct injury. Because of the laxity of the tissues and the venous plexi in the lower lid, it is usually more prominent there. When swelling of the upper lid alone develops within a few hours of injury, and when this is associated with edema over the forehead region, it implies that blood has seeped down from the subgaleal tissues into the upper eyelid. A direct injury may also lead to subconjunctival hemorrhages. The blood collects on either side of the cornea and is more obvious centrally, decreasing towards the periphery. After retro-orbital hemorrhage, which is frequently associated with fracture of the anterior fossa or of the malar bone, the blood may seep forward to appear first at the outer canthus. In a few hours, or after a day or so, it reaches the limbus where it stops and forms a sharp crescentic margin. Gravity tends to make the blood collect more in the lower than the upper half of the eye and this characteristic pyramidal-shaped hemorrhage is evidence of injury situated more posteriorly. Proptosis is frequently seen with frontal injuries and results either from bony displacement of the orbit or from hemorrhage within the orbit. Proptosis may also be a sign of a carotid-cavernous fistula. A bruit which is auscultated over the orbit is found with this lesion.

EYE SIGNS IN COMA

The evaluation of comatose patients requires several techniques which are routinely used in the neuro-ophthalmologic examination. Coma has been defined by Doctors Plum and Posner as "states in which psychological and motor responses to stimulation are either completely lost (deep coma) or reduced to only rudimentary reflex motor responses (moderately deep coma). " In evaluating the unconscious patient, the examining physician cannot obtain essential information which is ordinarily available from the mental and sensory examinations. An accurate history is important but, more often than not, the history must be obtained from relatives or other informants. Almost 40% of patients admitted for altered states of consciousness have a history of excessive alcohol or drug ingestion, and thus inquiry must be made as to the ingestion of narcotics or tranquilizers and especially anticoagulants. History of mental illness, head injury, seizures, or fainting spells, or the presence of heart disease, hypertension, kidney disease, diabetes, and cerebrovascular disease must be ascertained.

Careful inspection of the patient and his belongings may provide significant information as to etiology. This should include the presence of empty drug bottles. During the inspection of the patient, examination of the head may disclose contusions or lacerations of the scalp. Diffuse or focal edema of the scalp without lacerations sometimes suggests the presence of multiple underlying fractures produced by blunt instruments. An ecchymosis over the mastoid area (Battle's sign) is caused by a fracture of the temporal bone, and bilateral medial orbital ecchymoses ("racoon eyes") may suggest an anterior basal skull fracture. The nose and ears should be examined for the presence of blood or cerebrospinal fluid leakage. A clear glucose-containing fluid in the nose or ears is most likely cerebrospinal fluid and indicates a basal skull fracture.

Cerebral fat embolism may occur in a patient who has had no head injury or one in whom there have been multiple injuries, usually to the long bones, with considerable soft tissue injury. The presence of petechiae in the skin, especially over the shoulders and upper part of the chest, are common signs. Examination of the lower conjunctivae may reveal them here. This may also be present in the vessels of the optic fundi.

The general examination should be performed and note made of the attitude of the body. The position of rigid extension of the limbs and retraction of the head can be seen with severe infections of the nervous system and with subarachnoid hemorrhage. However, many patients with subarachnoid bleeding do not manifest meningeal signs during the first 24 to 48 hours.

Ophthalmoscopic examination is important because it provides an important reference from which later developments such as papilledema can be judged. Papilledema from increased intracranial pressure is rarely seen during the first 24 hours, although occasionally there may be a slight blurring of the optic disc margins or fullness of the veins. Examination for the presence of hemorrhage is essential. These are common in association with subarachnoid hemorrhage and are usually flame-shaped and lie adjacent to the optic disc. In severe cases a subhyloid hemorrhage may be seen. The state of the vessels should be noted particularly in patients suspected of having cerebrovascular disease. Massive vitreous hemorrhage or commotio-retinae may be the explanation for the finding of a fixed dilated pupil.

In performing the neuro-ophthalmologic examination, valuable information concerning the level of the brain involved, the nature of the involvement, and the prognosis can be obtained by evaluating (1) the size and reactivity of the pupils, (2) the eye movements, and (3) the vestibulo-ocular responses.

The afferent stimulus for the pupillary light reflex commences in the retinal ganglion cells, traverses the nerve fiber layer, and travels in the optic nerves accompanied by the retinal visual receptor axons through crossed and uncrossed pathways in the optic chiasm into the optic tracts. From the optic tracts the pathway turns medially anterior to the lateral geniculate body and enters the pretectal region. From these nuclei, fibers are connected bilaterally to the Edinger-Westphal nuclei. The efferent tract from the Edinger-Westphal nuclei traverses the oculomotor nerve and finally innervates the pupillary sphincter and ciliary body, after synapsing in the ciliary ganglion, via the inferior division of the oculomotor nerve. A helpful point to consider in examining an unconscious patient with a unilateral dilated and fixed pupil is to instill 2 drops of 2% pilocarpine into the eye. If the pupil was previously dilated with a mydriatic, the pilocarpine will have little, if any, effect on pupil size. If the pupil is dilated secondary to an internal ophthalmoplegia, the pupil will promptly and maximally constrict within 5 to 10 minutes. Unilateral absence of the direct and consensual light reflex indicates an efferent parasympathetic lesion of the oculomotor nerve on the ipsilateral side. Unilateral absence of the direct light reflex can be seen with pretectal lesions. Small, irregular pupils which do not respond to light, without evidence of oculomotor paralysis, are characteristic of central nervous system syphilis. This is occasionally also seen in patients with diabetes.

Midbrain damage can produce pupillary signs. Involvement of the dorsal region of the tectum or pretectum can interrupt the pupillary light reflex resulting in slightly widened, round, regular pupils that are fixed to light but spontaneously fluctuate in size and may show frequent oscillations with retention of the ciliospinal reflex. The diameter of the pupils is approximately 5 to 6 mm. The ciliospinal reflex consists of pupillary dilatation which is evoked by noxious cutaneous stimuli. This reflex produces ipsilateral mydriasis after pinching the neck. Painful stimuli of the face or trunk can also evoke the reaction and there may be a lesser degree of contralateral mydriasis as well.

The recognition of defects in function of the tectum by pupillary signs is significant in that small lesions in the midbrain tegmental area frequently involve the periaqueductal gray matter and cause loss of consciousness. Thus, the accompanying pupillary changes help in localizing the anatomic lesion.

Involvement of the nuclear region of the midbrain almost always causes interruption of the sympathetic and parasympathetic pathways to the eye. The pupils then are usually in midposition, 4-5mm in diameter, slightly irregular and often unequal, and unresponsive to all stimuli. This may occur with midbrain damage from transtentorial herniation, neoplasms, granulomas, and infarctions.

Lesions involving the oculomotor nerves between their nuclei and point of emergence from the brainstem can produce a total ophthalmoplegia with involvement of the pupil. Such oculomotor palsies are frequently bilateral, in contrast to peripheral third nerve palsies which are usually unilateral. A unilateral fixed pupil associated with outward deviation of the eye, with or without ptosis of the eyelid, indicates third nerve damage.

Lesions of the pontine tegmentum interrupt the descending sympathetic pathways and produce small pupils bilaterally. Pinpoint pupils may mean pontine hemorrhage and are thought to result from parasympathetic irritation in combination with sympathetic interruption. Involvement of the lateral portion of the medulla and the ventrolateral portion of the cervical spinal cord can produce a Horner's syndrome with slight ptosis and pupillary miosis, but the light reflex is not abolished. Peripheral lesions which affect either the third nerve or the sympathetic pathways can produce pupillary abnormalities. The pupillary fibers are susceptible when uncal herniation compresses the nerve against the posterior cerebral artery or the tentorium cerebelli. The pupillary dilatation may then precede extraocular muscle abnormalities. The third nerve may be compressed in this manner by an aneurysm of the posterior communicating artery. Rarely, lesions compressing the third nerve near its origin in the midbrain can produce an oculomotor palsy without pupillary dilatation. The pupil on the side of an occluded carotid artery, causing infarction of the cerebral hemisphere, may be constricted. This is thought to result from damage to the sympathetic fibers which surround the carotid artery, from a decrease in blood flow through the vasa nervorum.

The preservation of the pupillary light reflex despite respiratory depression, decerebrate rigidity, motor flaccidity, or absence of the vestibulo-ocular response suggests metabolic coma. If anoxia can be ruled out, the absence of the pupillary light reflex strongly implies that the disease is structural rather than metabolic. The pupillary responses must always be evaluated with magnification in a bright light.

The evaluation of ocular motility is also helpful in localizing the anatomic region involved in the production of coma. The anatomy of eye movements will be covered very briefly. Fibers from the gaze centers in the frontal cortex, mediating voluntary eye movements, and the occipital cortex, related to visual fixation, descend through the internal capsule into the brainstem. Fibers controlling conjugate lateral gaze are thought to decussate in the brainstem posterior to the trochlear nucleus and synapse in the contralateral pons near the abducens nucleus. This region is thought to be the pontine paramedian reticular formation. Fibers controlling conjugate vertical gaze are thought to reach the oculomotor nuclei from the cerebral hemispheres, bilaterally, travelling through the regions of the pretectal and posterior commissural nuclei.

Fibers of the medial longitudinal fasciculus interconnect the oculomotor, trochlear, and abducens nuclei. This pathway lies anterior to the periaqueductal gray matter. Fibers from the semi-circular canals of the inner ear and the fastigial nucleus of the cerebellum synapse in the vestibular nuclei and traverse the medial longitudinal fasciculus to innervate the ocular nuclei and thus connect the semicircular canals and cerebellum with the eye muscles. The major vestibular pathways go to the contralateral abducens nucleus and to the ipsilateral and contralateral oculomotor nuclei. Fibers mediating proprioception from the neck muscles reach the oculomotor nuclei via the medial longitudinal fasciculus which descends into the cervical spinal cord to the level of C-2 or C-3.

In a comatose patient with intact brainstem oculomotor function, the eyes often move spontaneously, showing slow, random, horizontal deviations. These movements can fluctuate in the same patient from conjugate to dysconjugate. These roving eye movements will disappear if brainstem function becomes further depressed.

Several types of nystagmus may be noted in patients with coma. Retractory nystagmus consists of irregular jerks of the eyes backward into the orbit, suggesting simultaneous contraction of all the extraocular muscles. This phenomenon accompanies lesions of the tegmentum of the midbrain. Convergence nystagmus consists of spontaneous slow drifting ocular divergence followed by a quick convergent movement. This may alternate with retractory nystagmus and also reflects a lesion of the midbrain. Ocular bobbing consists of episodes of intermittent, conjugate, rapid, downward movements which are followed by return to the primary position. This occurs with destructive lesions of the caudal pons. Nystagmoid jerking of a single eye in either the horizontal, vertical, or rotary direction also can be found with severe midpontine or lower pontine disease.

It should be noted that in a comatose patient with intact extraocular muscle pathways, the eyes are directed straight ahead. Deviation of either eye more than a few degrees from this physiologic position of rest usually indicates abnormal extraocular muscle function.

Conditions which produce coma cause one of three types of abnormal conjugate lateral gaze. The first is a temporary loss of contraversion when a lesion in one cerebral hemisphere disrupts supranuclear cerebral pathways. The eyes thus will deviate conjugately to the innervated side, or the side of the lesion. There is also associated contralateral hemiparesis so the eyes "look" at the normal arm and leg. Nystagmus is absent. The second abnormality is caused by an irritative phenomenon which causes the eyes to deviate away from the cerebral lesion. This contraversion of the eyes is seen with cerebral hemorrhage and is then replaced by the deviation of the eyes to the side of the lesion. Contraversion of the eyes associated with status epilepticus has a jerking, nystagmoid, and clonic character similar to that of motor seizures. Lesions in the pons which involve the supranuclear oculomotor fibers below the decussation can produce conjugate ocular deviation in which the eyes cannot be brought past the midline toward the lesion and thus spontaneously deviate away from the lesion. If the lesion is also affecting the corticospinal pathway, the hemiparesis is contralateral to the lesion so that the eyes "look" at the paralyzed side. Thus, involuntary conjugate deviation of the eyes toward a normal arm and leg suggests a hemispheric lesion and if the deviation is toward a paralyzed arm and leg, a pontine brainstem lesion.

Dysconjugate positions of the eyes result when nuclear or infranuclear oculomotor pathways in the brainstem are damaged. Lesions involving the oculomotor nucleus, or nerve, cause the involved eye to deviate outward. If the oculomotor lesion is in the brainstem, the pupil is dilated, at least to some degree, and light fixed. If the oculomotor lesion is in the peripheral fibers, the pupil is usually, but not always, dilated. With unilateral abducens paralysis, the eyes converge. In very deep coma, the pre-existing dysconjugate gaze may disappear since the innervation has been removed from the oculomotor muscles and the eyes assume the physiologic position of rest.

Abnormalities of upward gaze also imply a brainstem lesion. Paralysis of upward gaze results from the lesion compressing or destroying the pretectal and posterior commissure region at the junction of the diencephalon and midbrain. Bilateral lesions of the medial longitudinal fasciculus can also produce defects in upward gaze. In the state of light coma, upward gaze can be examined by holding the lid open and stimulating the cornea. This will result in lid closure and upward deviation of the eyes. Deviation of the eyes below the horizontal meridian also reflects brainstem dysfunction, most often involving the midbrain tectum. Resting vertical dysconjugate gaze implies a lesion of the internuclear or supranuclear pathways. In skew deviation, one eye is hypotropic and adducted and the other is hypertropic and abducted.

Two techniques which are valuable in the neuro-ophthalmologic evaluation of unresponsive states include the oculocephalic (doll's head) and vestibulo-ocular reflexes. These techniques are valuable in determining (1) whether the unresponsive state is psychogenic or organic, (2) the depth or stage of unconsciousness, as well as (3) the integrity of the extraocular movements.

In the normal, awake subject, the oculocephalic reflex consists of conjugate deviation of the eyes while fixing a target and turning the head. Rapid passive turning of the head results in contralateral conjugate deviation of the eyes opposite to the head movement. Rapid flexion and extension of the head will also result in opposite vertical deviation of the eyes. In an unresponsive patient the eyelids are held open and the head is rapidly turned to one side and then to the other. If the eyes are observed to move conjugately opposite to the head movements, the reflex is intact. This reflex is present in lighter states of unconsciousness and will disappear in deeper stages. When the reflex is absent, the eyes do not move from the midposition despite the change in head position. Nystagmus may be elicited on lateral gaze and provides a clue to brainstem dysfunction. In addition, an oculocephalic reflex which is intact in one direction and absent in the other direction suggests paralysis of conjugate gaze to one side. This is usually associated with a brain-stem lesion or ocular nerve paresis. One eye may abduct while the other eye remains in the midposition suggesting the presence of the syndrome of internuclear ophthalmoplegia.

The vestibulo-ocular reflex is elicited by positioning the head 30° above the horizontal so that the lateral semicircular canal is verti-cal and thus stimulation can evoke a maximal response. After as-certaining that the tympanic membrane is intact, cool water at 30° centigrade is introduced into the external canal for 3 minutes until approximately 200 cc have entered. In the normal, awake person, the characteristic response is a coarse horizontal nystagmus with the rapid component away from the irrigated ear and most pro-nounced on gaze in the direction opposite the side of stimulation. The rapid component of the nystagmus is in the direction away from the side of stimulation and the slow component is toward the side of stimulation. In addition, in the awake patient, there is veering and past-pointing to the side of stimulation. Nausea and vomiting may also ensue.

In states of unresponsiveness, there may be four responses on ca-loric stimulation. In stage one, caloric irrigation evokes the re-sponse seen in the awake patient; in stage two, cold calorics pro-duce tonic conjugate deviation of the eyes to the side of stimulation with a fine nystagmus. In stage three, the cold calorics will produce tonic conjugate deviation of the eyes to the side of stimulation with-out nystagmus. In stage four, the cold calorics produce no ocular response, the eyes remaining in or near the midposition.

In order to test vertical eye movements, both auditory canals can be irrigated simultaneously with cold water. The eyes will deviate downward. When warm water at 44° centigrade is used, the eyes will deviate upward.

The presence of an internuclear ophthalmoplegia may be suspected when the eye ipsilateral to the lesion fails to adduct on caloric irri-gation. Since an isolated medial rectus weakness is very rare, the reflex failure of one or both eyes to adduct is probably diagnostic of internuclear ophthalmoplegia.

In the foregoing discussion of the neuro-ophthalmologic evaluation of the comatose patient, the term coma has been used as a general-ization to include causes of unresponsiveness.

It should be mentioned that the abnormal pupillary and oculomotor signs, which have been described as occurring with impaired states of consciousness, may also be found in the alert patient.

PAPILLEDEMA AND OPTIC NERVE DISEASE

The differentiation of papilledema from other causes which produce swelling or pallor of the optic nerve head is extremely important.

"Papilledema" is the term applied to swelling of the optic disc that results from increased intracranial pressure. "Edema of the optic disc" refers to swelling of the disc which is of local or systemic origin. There are causes of blurring of the optic disc as well as edema of the disc which are not associated with increased intra-cranial pressure. Hyaline bodies (drusen) produce elevation of the optic disc. In young children, the drusen may be deep in the nerve and not easily visible with the ophthalmoscope. However, with age, they become more easily visible, are refractile, and are confused less often with papilledema. Tilting of the optic disc, optic nerve pits, and membranes about the disc are developmental anomalies which may cause field defects and can be confused with papilledema. Myelinated nerve fibers can also mimic papilledema.

A list of the causes of papilledema, benign intracranial hyperten-sion, and pseudopapilledema, are found in Tables 2 and 3.

Many theories have been entertained regarding the pathogenesis of papilledema. Perhaps the most valid one is that obstruction of the venous return from the eye in conjunction with other factors may be the cause of papilledema. The earliest sign of papilledema is hy-peremia of the disc which is secondary to capillary dilatation. Ven-ous distension ensues and the A-V ratio is increased. The optic cup begins to fill and there is then blurring of the optic disc margins. Blurring of the disc margin begins on the nasal side. An early sign which may precede the gross blurring of the disc margin is the de-velopment of Wises' lines on the temporal side of the disc. These are curved lines which are concentric with the disc and are the re-sult of peripapillary retinal displacement secondary to edema of the disc. The retina is thus thrown into folds and there are reflections from the internal limiting membrane. As the disc swells and ele-vation ensues, the vessels are displaced and curve over the edge of the disc as they travel towards the retina. The height of the papil-ledema can be measured from the highest point of the edema on the disc to the part of the retina which is flat.

The relationship of the diopters of elevation of actual anatomic ele-vation is about 3 diopters to 1 mm in a phakic person and 2 diopters to 1 mm in an aphakic person. Although approximately 40% of the normal population does not show a spontaneous venous pulse, if it is present, there is usually no significant elevation of intracranial pressure. If it is absent, no conclusions can be reached. Hemor-rhages are an indication of rapidity of onset of the papilledema, when they are the predominant feature. The hemorrhages of papilledema, secondary to increased intracranial pressure, are found in the pos-teria pole, while those associated with malignant hypertension or occlusion of the central retinal vein are present in the periphery as well as in the posterior pole. White, cotton-wool exudates are seen and are disposed of in a manner similar to the hemorrhages. The macular star represents exudates found in Henle's fiber layer and assumes its configuration. The presence of a macular star im-plies that the edema has been present for weeks or months. Vision is usually normal in papilledema secondary to increased intracran-ial pressure. As the papilledema becomes chronic, optic atrophy ensues and vision may become impaired.

252/ Neuro-Ophthalmologic Emergencies

I. INCREASED INTRACRANIAL PRESSURE
A. Brain tumors - particularly tumors of cerebellum, fourth ventricle, meningioma of anterior and middle cranial fossae, pinealoma, craniopharyngioma, metastatic, glioblastoma
B. Benign intracranial hypertension (pseudotumor cerebri)
1. Intracranial venous thromboses (sagittal, straight or lateral sinuses, vein of Galen)
2. Disorders of endocrine glands
a. Adrenal (Addison's disease, Cushing's syndrome)
b. Ovarian (menstrual dysfunction, obesity, pregnancy, menarche, contraceptive agents)
c. Parathyroid-hypoparathyroidism
3. Vitamin and drug therapy
a. Vitamin A
b. Tetracyclines
c. Nalidixic acid
C. Brain abscess (temporal lobe and cerebellum)
D. Subarachnoid hemorrhage
E. Subdural hematoma
F. Hydrocephalus
G. Meningitis
H. Postmeningitis and arachnoiditis
I. Craniostenosis

II. DISEASE OF THE ORBIT
A. Tumors of optic nerve
B. Thyroid ophthalmopathy

III. OCULAR PATHOLOGY
A. Acute glaucoma
B. Hypotony - secondary to trauma, surgery, uveitis

IV. SYSTEMIC DISEASE
A. Malignant hypertension
B. Blood dyscrasias
C. Anemia
D. Hypovolemia
E. Pulmonary insufficiency
F. Guillain-Barre syndrome (infectious polyneuritis)
G. Poliomyelitis
H. Lead poisoning
I. Sarcoidosis

TABLE 3

CAUSES OF PSEUDOPAPILLEDEMA

1. Myelinated nerve fibers
2. "Gliosis" - Remnants of Bergmeister's papilla
3. Hyperopia
4. Hyaline bodies (drusen)
5. Crescents (congenital, myopic)
6. Dysversion of disc
7. Colobomas
8. Retrolental fibroplasia
9. Neoplasms of disc

The nonocular symptoms of increased intracranial pressure include headache, vomiting, circulatory and respiratory disturbances, and psychic changes (Table 4).

TABLE 4

SIGNS OF INCREASED INTRACRANIAL PRESSURE

A. Nonocular symptoms of increased intracranial pressure
   1. Headache
   2. Vomiting
   3. Circulatory and respiratory disturbances
   4. Psychic changes
B. Ocular signs of increased intracranial pressure
   1. Papilledema
   2. Nonspecific ocular paresis (especially of abducens nerve)
   3. Clivus ridge syndrome (pupillary disturbances)
   4. Bilateral exophthalmos - occasionally

Headache may be one of the earlier symptoms of increased intracranial pressure. In some cases the headache may be increased by coughing and straining. Vomiting, bradycardia, and difficulty in respiration may be secondary to irritation of the medullary centers. The ocular signs of increased intracranial pressure include papilledema, ocular pareses (particularly of the abducens nerve), the clivus ridge syndrome (pupillary disturbances) and, occasionally, bilateral exophthalmos (Table 4). The increase in intracranial pressure results in compression of the sixth nerve. Loss of consciousness and motor rigidity may occur secondary to compression, and motor rigidity may occur secondary to compression of the cerebral cortex and the reduction of its blood supply. Tentorial herniation can produce pressure on the cerebral peduncles accounting for the muscular rigidity and can compress the third nerve, producing dilatation of the pupils. Transient blurring of vision may occur lasting approximately 15 to 30 seconds. These obscurations of vision secondary to papilledema are brief compared to the unilateral loss of vision secondary to carotid artery insufficiency which usually last from 5 to 10 minutes. Visual acuity between the episodes of obscuration is usually normal. This provides a differentiating factor between papilledema and optic neuritis. In optic neuritis there is pronounced loss of vision. With chronic papilledema there may be a gradual loss of vision. Enlargement of the blind spot may be the only demonstrable field change. Concentric contraction of the peripheral fields for form and colors is present during the late stages of papilledema. The nasal field will suffer more than the temporal field. There may be progressive narrowing which continues until only a small temporal island remains. This island may surround the blind spot and when it alone remains the patient may be completely without vision and the pupils are dilated and do not respond to light. The concentric contraction of the peripheral field mentioned above is usually present when optic atrophy is noted.

Intravenous fluorescein is very useful in the detection of early stages of papilledema and the differentiation from elevated structural anomalies that closely resemble papilledema. Fluorescence does not persist in the capillaries of the normal disc even if its margins are blurred or if it is anomalously elevated. If the disc blurring is the result of capillary stasis secondary to papilledema, fluorescein will fill these capillaries and will leak into the extra-vascular tissues. The disc will then stain for more than 10 minutes.

Optic neuritis is the term used to denote involvement of the optic nerve as a result of inflammation, demyelination, or degeneration. Papillitis indicates neuritis of the ophthalmoscopically visible portion of the optic nerve. It is characterized by swelling of the optic disc and is an anteriorly situated form of optic neuritis. An optic neuroretinitis signifies a papillitis plus involvement of the retina. Retrobulbar neuritis refers to a neuritis located behind the lamina cribrosa so that at its onset it is not visible ophthalmoscopically. Optic neuritis must be differentiated from conditions which cause the optic discs to appear elevated and from conditions which cause loss of vision without elevation of the disc. Papilledema has already been considered above. Pseudopapilledema is characterized by blurring of the optic disc margins and elevation of the disc. The blind spots may also be enlarged. However, the veins are not engorged, the capillaries on the optic disc are not dilated, and there are no hemorrhages or exudates adjacent to the disc. The elevation appears solid and not edematous. The vessels do not appear to dip into a ring of edema but, instead, ride over the papilla. Hyaline bodies in the tissue of the optic disc are considered to be the major cause of pseudopapilledema. Any type of refractive error may be present, although the condition is more commonly associated with higher hyperopic or astigmatic errors. Fundus photography and intravenous fluorescein angiography are helpful in evaluating doubtful cases. In papillitis or retrobulbar neuritis, there is usually a decrease of visual acuity and impairment of the visual field.

The most common visual field defect is a unilateral centrocecal or central scotoma, but any type of field defect may be present, including an arcuate defect with or without retention of good visual acuity, a scotoma breaking through to the periphery, or total loss of vision. Pain on movement and tenderness on palpation of the globe is common with papillitis and retrobulbar neuritis. In Table 5, a list of the causes of optic neuropathy is included, along with a differential diagnosis of unilateral and bilateral optic neuropathy. Papilledema is more frequently bilateral, whereas papillitis is more commonly unilateral. The ophthalmoscopic appearance of papilledema and papillitis may be exactly the same. Careful examination of the pupillary reactions is important in the diagnosis of optic nerve disease. Optic neuritis with good visual acuity is not uncommon and is often mistaken for papilledema. The type of optic neuritis with normal visual acuity can be diagnosed by the presence of a Marcus-Gunn pupillary phenomenon, a nerve fiber bundle visual field defect, and cells in the vitreous on slit-lamp examination.

When visual acuity has been reduced, even as poor as to only light perception, improvement may commence within one to four weeks. However, this improvement may be delayed for several months. Moreover, permanent blindness or poor vision may ensue. A papillitis has a poorer prognosis for return of vision than a retrobulbar neuritis. In a retrobulbar neuritis there is practically no evidence of edema or inflammation of the optic nerve head. Following a papillitis, a secondary optic atrophy may develop in which the disc margins become indistinct because there is glial tissue formation on the disc. In addition, the retinal arteries become narrow. When the optic neuritis has involved the optic nerve posterior to the entrance of the central retinal artery into the nerve, pallor may develop, but usually the retinal vessels remain normal.

Optic atrophy is the sequela of any process which causes shrinkage of cells and fibers and an over-all diminution in size of the optic nerve. It is caused by a pathologic process which has produced degeneration of axones in the retinogeniculate pathway.

Papilledema may be the general effect of elevated intracranial pressure having no localizing significance, may be associated with no neurologic abnormality, or can be indicative of a potentially fatal neurologic disease. The treatment of papilledema consists of determining the cause of the increased intracranial pressure or the cause of the edema of the optic nerve, if increased intracranial pressure is not present. The aid of a neurologist or neurosurgeon should be sought in the performance of the detailed neurologic evaluation which should include the clinical neurologic examination, an electroencephalogram, skull series, and a radioactive isotope study. If any of these evaluations are abnormal, hospitalization and further contrast studies would be indicated. The causes of pseudopapilledema are usually not progressive but it is occasionally difficult to differentiate between papilledema and pseudopapilledema.

Multiple sclerosis is probably the most common cause of optic neuritis in patients below the age of 45, accounting for approximately 20% in children, and 20-40% in adults. This is characterized by acute unilateral retrobulbar neuritis with a tendency to improve within 4 to 6 weeks. There is as yet no established treatment for multiple sclerosis. Steroids are used extensively at the present

TABLE 5

CAUSES OF OPTIC NEUROPATHY

I. INFLAMMATION
   A. Intraocular
   B. Orbital
   C. Sinusitis
   D. Meningitis
   E. Systemic

II. DEMYELINATING
   A. Multiple sclerosis
   B. Neuromyelitis optica
   C. Postviral
   D. Schilder's disease
   E. Carcinomatosis

III. METABOLIC
   A. Diabetes
   B. Vitamin deficiency
      1. Pernicious anemia
      2. Parasitic disease of G. I. tract
      3. Pellagra
      4. Beriberi
   C. Neuropathy of pregnancy and lactation
   D. Thyroid ophthalmopathy

IV. HEREDITARY
   A. Leber's disease
   B. Hereditary CNS disease

V. VASCULAR DISEASE AND ISCHEMIC NEUROPATHY (PERI-ARTERITIS, TEMPORAL ARTERITIS, ATHEROSCLEROTIC OCCLUSIVE VASCULAR DISEASE)

VI. GENERALIZED NONINFECTIOUS DISEASE
   A. Blood dyscrasias
   B. Blood loss: Sudden hypotension or secondary anemia
   C. Allergy - chocolate, fish, pork, turkey, poison ivy, tetanus antitoxin, vaccines, bee sting
   D. Sarcoidosis

VII. NUTRITIONAL
   A. Alcoholism
   B. Tobacco

VIII. TOXIC
   A. Drugs
   B. Poisons

IX. TUMORS
   A. Lymphoma
   B. Metastatic
   C. Glioma

time. It is agreed that they have no significant effect on the ultimate course of the disease but it is maintained that their administration will lessen the severity and shorten the length of an acute episode, particularly an attack of retrobulbar neuritis. Adequate nutrition with the addition of vitamin supplements and the prevention or prompt treatment of intercurrent infections are important. It has been estimated that 20 to 50% of the patients with retrobulbar neuritis, with onset between the ages of 20 to 45 years, will develop signs of multiple sclerosis within 10 to 15 years. Involvement of the optic nerve in multiple sclerosis may occur in a subacute or chronic form with diminution of visual acuity and various types of visual field defects or scotomas. The optic disc in patients with a chronic optic neuritis or in patients with a history of previous retrobulbar neuritis may appear smaller than normal and there may be pallor of the optic nerve head, especially temporal pallor. Optic atrophy was found in 11% and temporal pallor in 65% (unilateral in 30% and bilateral in 35%), of 45 cases which were proved at autopsy at Montefiore Hospital.

Neuromyelitis optica is suggested by an acute bilateral optic neuritis which is followed or preceded by a transverse myelitis. There may be complete, or almost complete, loss of vision. Occasionally, a bilateral optic neuritis may occur without myelitis and it is not known whether this represents a form of neuromyelitis optica.

In Leber's disease, the onset of poor vision can occur at any age and males are more commonly afflicted than females. The signs and symptoms can be the same as a bilateral optic neuritis from the causes listed above. A family history must be present to establish specifically this diagnosis. The possibility that the optic atrophy is associated with other central nervous system disorders must be considered.

In patients above the age of 50, the most common cause of optic nerve disease is vascular. The nutrient vessels of the optic nerves may be occluded secondary to hypertension, atherosclerosis, or an arteritis resulting in an ischemic optic neuritis. An erythrocyte sedimentation rate should be obtained in all patients above the age of 50 who present with the signs and symptoms of an optic neuritis.

In evaluating the causes of a bilateral optic neuritis, a complete blood count should always be obtained, as well as specialized tests for the presence of vitamin B-12 deficiency. Secondary anemias, leukemias, as well as polycythemia vera can produce an optic neuritis. The optic neuritis secondary to blood loss produces visual impairment by the sudden hypotension which results, or by the secondary anemia if the blood loss is progressive. An investigation for the causes of blood loss should be performed.

Metabolic disorders such as those found with diabetes mellitus or thyroid disease can produce optic neuritis. Nutritional optic neuropathy is thought to be the most common cause of bilateral centrocecal scotomas. This is found with alcoholism and is probably the mechanism in tobacco amblyopia as well. With a toxic amblyopia, the pupils react to light although vision is impaired. This can occur with carbon monoxide intoxication. Other causes of toxic amblyopia include anoxia, carbon tetrachloride, chloromycetin, dilantin, marijuana, quinine, and salicylates.

Malignant lymphomas can produce lesions in the optic nerve. Metastatic tumors and meningiomas are found more frequently in adults and the optic gliomas usually affect children. A slowly progressive unilateral loss of vision which is accompanied by proptosis and enlargement of the optic foramen suggests the presence of a tumor.

OPTIC CHIASM

Visual symptoms are conspicuous with lesions in the region of the optic chiasm and may be the only symptoms. This may include visual field defects, loss of visual acuity, and optic atrophy which may be variable and delayed. Bitemporal hemianopia is considered the characteristic field defect of a chiasmal lesion. However, there may also be partial temporal hemianopias, unilateral blindness with contralateral depression of the superior temporal quadrant, irregular altitudinal and asymmetric scotomas, as well as bilateral paracentral scotomas. Central scotomas in one or both eyes resulting in loss of visual acuity can also result from a chiasmal lesion. Hallucinations, headaches, and oculomotor palsies can all be found with involvement of the optic chiasm. If the hypothalamus is implicated, the syndrome of diabetes insipidus can ensue consisting of polydipsia and polyuria. With further involvement of the hypothalamus, there may be mental changes as well as drowsiness and signs of hypopituitarism.

Characteristic x-ray changes of disease of the optic chiasm include enlargement of the sella turcica, erosion of the clinoid processes, calcification within or above the sella, hyperostosis of the tuberculum sellae, hyperostosis of the lesser wing of the sphenoid, and enlargement of the optic foramen.

The region of the optic chiasm may be involved in multiple sclerosis, diffuse sclerosis with meningitis, and chiasmic arachnoiditis.

One of four of all intracranial tumors is said to arise in the region of the optic chiasm and visual symptoms may constitute the initial manifestation. The tumors include the pituitary adenoma, craniopharyngioma and suprasellar meningioma. Aneurysms may cause a bitemporal hemianopia with signs of panhypopituitarism and enlargement of the sella turcica. The signs which suggest aneurysm in contradistinction to adenoma include supraorbital pain, episodes of intense headache, sudden blindness in one eye with a temporal field defect in the other eye, anesthesia in the region of one eye, and unilateral ophthalmoplegia. The chromophobe adenoma is the most frequent pituitary tumor which presents with visual symptoms. The most characteristic x-ray finding is enlargement of the sella turcica. With a craniopharyngioma, there may be suprasellar calcification.

The suprasellar meningioma may give rise to visual symptoms only and may be overlooked. Injury to the optic chiasm with a bitemporal hemianopia occurs with fractures of the base of the skull.

The characteristics of the monocular syndrome of incipient prechiasmal optic nerve compression are a slowly progressing dimming of vision with near normal visual acuity, poor color perception, a Marcus-Gunn pupillary sign, and a normal appearance of the optic disc. In the presence of these findings, one should resort to polytomography of the sella and optic canals, pneumotomography, and selective angiography with subtraction and magnification, in order to arrive at a diagnosis.

Pituitary apoplexy is a syndrome characterized by intense headaches, unilateral or bilateral ophthalmoplegia, and the sudden occurrence of blindness in both eyes, and coma. Without surgical intervention death may ensue in hours or days. This syndrome usually develops as a result of hemorrhage into a pituitary adenoma or an infarction within such a tumor.

CEREBROVASCULAR DISEASE (Table 6)

Occlusive disease of the carotid and vertebrobasilar arteries may frequently produce visual signs and symptoms. These signs and symptoms are caused by local tissue ischemia of the eye or of the visual pathways.

TABLE 6

SIGNS AND SYMPTOMS OF CEREBROVASCULAR DISEASE OF INTEREST TO THE OPHTHALMOLOGIST

1. Amaurosis fugax
2. Unilateral loss of vision caused by occlusion of a central retinal artery, of one of its branches, or of the artery to the optic nerve
3. Binocular visual defects secondary to occlusion of a middle cerebral artery or its branches with resulting incongruous homonymous hemianopia
4. Binocular visual defects secondary to occlusion of a posterior cerebral artery with resulting congruous homonymous hemianopia
5. Hypotensive manifestations in the retina on the affected side, including cotton-wool patches in the retina, widening of the arterioles and venules, and venous-stasis retinopathy
6. Hemorrhagic glaucoma
7. Bright embolic cholesterol plaques in the retinal arterioles
8. Lowering of the ipsilateral retinal artery pressure
9. Horner's syndrome

Blood flow to a given area, which has been partially compromised by an atherosclerotic process in the local circulation, can be further impaired by hypotension, decreased cardiac output, vasospasm, transient failure of the collateral circulation or narrowing of the lumen of the extracranial vessels in the neck or thorax. The transient ischemic attack is a temporary episode of neurologic dysfunction which, when confined to the distribution of the carotid system, may produce transient blurring of vision, headaches, focal seizures, hemiplegia, hemisensory defects, and aphasia. The ocular hallmark of occlusive carotid disease is amaurosis fugax (fleeting blindness) in which the patient suddenly loses vision in one eye, which lasts up to 10 minutes and then gradually returns. Amaurosis fugax may be total or partial in that the dimming of vision can occur in the upper or lower half of the field of vision, or the sensation may be that of specks of bright light fleeting across the field. The patient may describe a curtain or a shade which obscures part of the vision of one eye or transient total loss of vision. These episodes may include burning or watering of the involved eye, transient paresthesis of the medial brow and forehead in the distribution of the terminal branches of the ophthalmic artery, and peculiar feelings behind the eye preceding the "blackout." The mechanism producing monocular blindness relates to the presence of atheromatous disease of the carotid artery in the neck. With superimposed hypotension or vasoconstriction, local ischemia can ensue. Mural thrombi may be dislodged from plaques in the carotid vessels, causing transient signs, and then fragment and disappear in the blood stream. A frequent finding in patients with a history of amaurosis fugax is shiny, yellow particles within the lumen of a retinal arteriole, usually at a bifurcation. This is considered to be a cholesterol crystal. White, nonreflecting plugs of material may also be seen within the retinal vessels. These are thought to be composed of platelets and fibrin, as well as fats. Hollenhorst found that 30% of patients with cerebrovascular insufficiency had one or more orange, yellow, or copper-colored intraluminal plaques lodged at the bifurcation of the retinal arterioles. He also found that 20% of patients undergoing endarterectomy had such particles within the retinal vasculature and presumed that these were flakes of cholesterol that had been washed into the retinal vascular tree from ulcerating atheromatous lesions in the neck, usually a stenotic lesion at the bifurcation of the carotid artery. The transient ischemic attacks usually cease after the carotid becomes completely occluded. Vision may remain good if collateral circulation through the circle of Willis or the external carotid artery has been accomplished. Transient loss of vision can also be caused by a cardiac arrhythmia, giant cell arteritis, or hypertensive crisis with increased venous pressure and fluctuating retinal perfusion secondary to an impending central retinal vein occlusion or with intermittent elevations of intraocular pressure as in polycythemia vera, severe anemias or thrombocytosis, and secondary to embolization from valvular heart disease such as is found in rheumatic heart disease and subacute bacterial endocarditis.

Transient ischemic episodes involving the vertebrobasilar arterial system produce bilateral blurring or dimming of vision almost as frequently as vertigo. There may be episodic diplopia, oscillopsia, internuclear ophthalmoplegia, nystagmus, and extraocular muscle palsies. These signs and symptoms are secondary to ischemia of the brainstem. Ischemia in the distribution of the posterior cerebral arteries can produce transient homonymous hemianopsia or transient blindness bilaterally. The pupillary responses are usually retained. Causes of the transient vascular insufficiency include atheromatous occlusion, changes in cardiac output and regional blood flow, hypertensive vascular disease causing slow reactivity of the brainstem and cortical arterioles, anemia and polycythemia, microembolization, and atheromata in the vertebral or basilar arteries. In addition, mechanical factors which restrict the flow of blood in the vertebral arteries include that produced on head movement by cervical spondylosis and kinking and tortuosity and redundancy of the extracranial portion of the vertebral arteries. An isolated, homonymous hemianopsia of sudden onset is the hallmark of vascular disease in the occipital lobe, usually involving the posterior cerebral artery. Homonymous quadrantopias, homonymous scotomas, or constriction of one or both visual fields, may occur.

Aortic arch disease may produce symptoms related to the carotid and vertebrobasilar system, including ocular, cerebral, and brainstem signs.

As indicated above, occlusion or decreased perfusion of the internal carotid artery may result in ipsilateral decrease in vision, or decreased ophthalmic artery pressure and contralateral hemiplegia. Amaurosis fugax has been described above and is the most common symptom of carotid artery insufficiency, occurring in about 40% of the cases. It is nearly always absent in patients after a completed stroke. About 85% of the patients with amaurosis fugax have lower ophthalmic artery pressures on that side. It should be recalled that if the loss of vision lasts longer than 5 minutes, the occlusive process is in the retina or optic nerve. Amaurosis fugax, which consists of sudden contraction of the visual field of one eye, varying from altitudinal anopsia to complete loss of vision, is followed by the gradual return to normal within 4 to 5 minutes. With involvement of the middle cerebral artery or its branches, a contralateral hemiplegia results with motor deficit more pronounced in the upper extremities. This is associated frequently with a contralateral hemisensory defect, contralateral homonymous hemianopia, and aphasia, if the lesion is in the dominant cerebral hemisphere. With involvement of the anterior cerebral artery there is a contralateral hemiplegia and, occasionally, a hemisensory defect. The defect is greater in the lower extremity.

Eighty percent of the patients with involvement of the vertebrobasilar system manifest ocular signs and symptoms. When the posterior cerebral artery is involved, there may be blurred vision due to unilateral or bilateral visual field defects. This is frequently associated with a contralateral homonymous hemianopia and with a concomitant hemisensory deficit in some cases. When other branches of the basilar artery are involved, episodes of vertigo, blurred vision or diplopia occur. There may be bilateral involvement with crossed syndromes involving motor and sensory functions, slurred speech, and incoordination. Cranial nerve abnormalities are frequent as well as nystagmus, particularly in the vertical plane. The posterior inferior cerebellar artery or vertebral artery syndrome is characterized by defective sensation or the ipsilateral face and contralateral body. This is associated with ipsilateral palate and vocal cord paralysis, dysphagia, ipsilateral Horner's syndrome, ipsilateral ataxia, and nystagmus. Insufficiency in the superior cerebellar artery is characterized by ataxia and involuntary movements, as well as loss of pain and temperature sensation involving the contralateral half of the body including the face. When the anterior inferior cerebellar artery is involved, there may be ipsilateral impairment of hearing, facial paralysis, Horner's syndrome, and loss of touch on the face on the same side as the lesion, as well as impairment of pain and temperature in the contralateral arm and leg and, occasionally, the face. Nystagmus and ataxia may be present as well. Vertebral artery occlusion can produce episodes of vertigo with unsteadiness or falling. The syndrome of decreased blood flow through one or both posterior cerebral arteries with resulting homonymous hemianopia may also be present. Turning of the head and neck or carotid compression may induce nystagmus.

Spontaneous subarachnoid or intracerebral hemorrhage is characterized by an apoplectiform onset with severe headaches, which are usually suboccipital in location, accompanied by nausea, vomiting, lethargy, confusion, coma, or seizures. There may be stiff neck, tenderness of the globe, as well as pain on ocular movement, and severe low back pain.

There are several approaches to the treatment of cerebrovascular disease. These include surgical endarterectomy, long-term anticoagulant therapy, and observation and treatment of concomitant disease such as hypertension, cardiac arrhythmias, diabetes, or blood dyscrasias and inflammatory disease of the vessels.

Subdural hemorrhage results from tearing of small veins which bridge the subdural space. It is secondary to severe or minor injury to the head but can occur in association with blood dyscrasias or in the elderly person without a history of trauma or blood dyscrasia. The trauma may also have preceded the onset of neurologic complaints by several weeks. The symptoms of chronic subdural hematoma include headache, variation in the state of the sensorium, mental confusion, as well as papilledema. Papilledema may be present in 30 to 50% of the patients with subdural hematomas. Ipsilateral dilatation of the pupils is the most common and most important pupillary sign and is an urgent indication for surgical intervention. Other cranial nerve signs, including nystagmus and cranial nerve palsies, may occur secondary to compression of the brainstem. Skull films may indicate the presence of a midline shift of a calcified pineal gland and carotid arteriography will confirm the diagnosis.

Hemorrhage into the extradural space is usually secondary to a tear in the middle meningeal artery but in approximately 15% of the cases, the bleeding occurs from one of the dural sinuses. The patient may lose consciousness at the time of trauma, which is then followed by a lucid interval of several hours with a subsequent relapse into coma accompanied by the development of hemiplegia. The initial coma is due to concussion or cerebral trauma and the secondary loss of consciousness and hemiplegia is the result of compression of the brain by expansion of the hemorrhage. The lucid interval may be absent in approximately 50% of the patients. In the usual case, the signs of brain compression, coma, and hemiplegia develop a few hours after the accident. However, this may be delayed for up to three weeks. On funduscopy, the optic discs are usually normal in patients who develop signs of cerebral compression within a few hours after injury. Papilledema may develop in patients who live from two to three weeks after the injury. The finding of a dilated pupil, which does not react to light or accommodation, accompanied by other signs of oculomotor palsy, is on the same side as the clot and is secondary to compression of the third nerve by the hippocampal gyrus which has herniated over the free edge of the tentorium. Extradural hemorrhage is the most fatal complication of head injury, with a mortality of 100% in untreated cases and over 50% in the treated cases. Immediate arteriography is necessary and is followed by surgical intervention.

TEMPORAL ARTERITIS

Temporal arteritis is a disease of the elderly, characterized by headache with sudden onset of blindness. Histologically, there are changes in the tunica media characterized by marked cellular infiltration, the presence of giant cells, and disintegration of the internal elastic lamina. There may be hyperplasia of the tunica intima with resulting obliteration of the lumen. There may also be involvement of the cerebral or cardiac vessels as well as the arteries of the limbs and gastrointestinal tract. Temporal arteritis is uncommon below the age of 60 years, almost 80% of the patients being above the age of 70. The disease is characterized by an initial phase of general malaise and weakness, myalgias, loss of appetite and weight, headache and insomnia. Pain in the jaws on chewing is frequent. The patient may complain of pain in the region of the eye or ear and the pain often follows the distribution of the superficial temporal artery. In a series of 175 patients with temporal arteritis, 37 presented with blindness. The visual symptoms are ischemic in origin and are related to an inflammatory arteritis of the ophthalmic artery and posterior ciliary vessels. The characteristic finding is engorgement and tenderness of the superficial temporal arteries on the side involved. The area about the superficial temporal arteries may be erythematous. Bruits have been described over the carotid arteries, the superficial temporal artery, as well as the orbit. Orbital bruits may be present before the blindness occurs. The erythrocyte sedimentation rate is markedly elevated and there is usually elevation of the alpha-1 and alpha-2 globulin fractions. Biopsy of the superficial temporal artery is necessary to confirm the diagnosis. However, the absence of a positive temporal artery biopsy does not contradict the diagnosis.

Blindness, in one or both eyes, may develop in patients with temporal arteritis, secondary to ischemia of the optic nerve or retina. In the natural course of the disease, about one-half of the patients are likely to become blind in one or both eyes. Blindness is unlikely to occur later than six months after the onset of the headache and usually occurs a few weeks following the headaches. Rarely, blindness may be the first manifestation of arteritis without any headaches. In the majority of the patients there is a slight or moderate swelling of the optic nerve head. There may be flame-shaped hemorrhages and cotton-wool exudates but little evidence of narrowing of the retinal arteries. The severity of the visual loss is usually out of proportion to the visible changes in the fundus. This observation is also seen in retrobulbar neuritis and compression of the optic nerve, in angiomas and aneurysms. The optic disc edema subsides within a few weeks and is replaced by optic atrophy with relatively normal retinal vessels. The ophthalmic ciliary arteries have been noted to be most severely involved by the arteritis and the central retinal artery is infrequently involved. Ophthalmoplegia is a less common manifestation of temporal arteritis, occurring in about 15% of the patients, usually during the active phase of the arteritis following the headache. There may be a palsy of the 3rd or 6th cranial nerve, with sparing of the pupil. This may be unilateral or bilateral. Diplopia may be present without overt evidence of an ocular palsy. The extraocular muscle palsies have a better prognosis than the visual impairment and complete or partial resolution is usual over a period of several months. The giant cell arteritis may involve the internal carotid and vertebral arteries, leading to occlusion of these vessels. The findings would be similar to those described above in the section on occlusive disease of the cerebral vasculature. Involvement of the skeletal musculature may be the cause of the so-called "polymyalgia rheumatica." This is characterized by pain and stiffness involving the muscles of the shoulders and thighs.

As stated above, the confirmatory tests include an elevated E. S. R. and a biopsy of the superficial temporal artery. The disease tends to run a course of several months to a year with the potential for blindness in one-half of the cases. Early treatment is essential and represents a medical emergency. Once there is evidence of an elevated E. S. R., immediate steroid therapy, 60 mg of prednisone daily, must be administered. This dosage can be reduced gradually after two to three weeks, but treatment must be continued for at least six months in order to prevent recurrence of symptoms or a rise in the E. S. R. Unfortunately, blindness can ensue even following the institution of steroid therapy. The blindness may be in the contralateral eye and not in the eye which is clinically involved.

ANEURYSMS AND ARTERIOVENOUS MALFORMATIONS

The most common cause of bleeding into the subarachnoid space is rupture of the meningeal vessels following trauma to the head.

Hemorrhage into the subarachnoid space may occur in patients with blood dyscrasias, intracranial tumors, angiomas, toxic or infectious diseases of the nervous system, and intracerebral hemorrhage. Bleeding into the subarachnoid space may also follow rupture of an aneurysm of one of the vessels in the subarachnoid space.

Intracranial aneurysms, ruptured or unruptured, are found in approximately 2% of all the autopsies performed in adults. Approximately 6 to 10% of all cerebrovascular lesions are due to rupture of an intracranial aneurysm.

The size of an aneurysm may vary. Aneurysms do not cause any pathologic changes in the nervous system unless they are so situated that they compress the cranial nerves. In approximately 25% of the cases, the aneurysms are multiple.

Intracranial aneurysms of the ophthalmic artery are rare. Because they are located adjacent to the optic nerve, these aneurysms may produce signs of optic nerve compression that mimic the symptoms of a retrobulbar neuritis. The usual signs and symptoms include a scotoma in one eye that progresses to loss of the nasal field on the involved side. Later on, there may be an upper temporal depression of the contralateral field and finally, blindness on the side of the aneurysm. The temporal field defect in the contralateral eye is caused by compression of the chiasm by the aneurysm. There may be erosion of the anterior clinoid processes and the intracranial portion of the optic canal on x-ray.

Infraclinoid aneurysms include those situated in the carotid artery within the cavernous sinus, as well as adjacent to the sella. This may produce a unilateral ophthalmoplegia, particularly involving the third nerve, but also the sixth and fourth nerve depending upon the portion of the cavernous sinus which is involved. There is intense pain in the area of distribution of the first, second, and third branches of the trigeminal nerve associated with hypesthesia in this area. The patient may complain of a sudden violent headache. Radiographically, there may be destruction in the region of the lesser wing of the sphenoid bone as well as the clinoid processes. The superior orbital fissure may be enlarged. With the posterior syndrome of the cavernous sinus, there is predominantly a sixth nerve palsy associated with involvement of the first, second, and third branches of the trigeminal nerve. In the so-called "middle syndrome," there is a complete ophthalmoplegia with involvement of the first and second branches of the trigeminal nerve, while in the anterior syndrome, there is involvement of the third cranial nerve or a complete ophthalmoplegia with findings predominantly in the first division of the trigeminal nerve. A so-called "intrasellar aneurysm of the internal carotid artery" within the cavernous sinus, may produce the chiasmal syndrome with an asymmetric bitemporal hemianopia and fluctuations in the character of the field defect as well as an ophthalmoplegia. Signs of trigeminal nerve involvement are absent but the patient still complains of severe headaches.

Supraclinoid aneurysms are caused by an aneurysm of the anterior cerebral and anterior communicating arteries. These are characterized by an atypical chiasmal syndrome with a bitemporal inferior quadrantanopia, unilateral or bilateral loss of vision, and fluctuations in the field defect as well as the visual acuity. The trigeminal nerve is not involved but there may be evidence of compression of the olfactory nerve. The field defect is rather sudden in onset, and the acute loss of vision may precede the full-blown signs of the subarachnoid hemorrhage.

An aneurysm at the junction of the carotid and posterior communicating artery is characterized by the sudden appearance of a unilateral headache, pain in the forehead or the eye, and the simultaneous appearance of a partial or complete oculomotor palsy with or without mydriasis and disturbance of accommodation. The pain is characteristically in the distribution of the ophthalmic branch of the trigeminal nerve. Frequently, the picture of so-called "ophthalmoplegic migraine" may be simulated by such an aneurysm.

An aneurysm of the posterior cerebral artery is quite rare and may produce an homonymous hemianopia. A third nerve palsy with a contralateral hemiplegia similar to that present in occlusive vascular disease can occur before the rupture of the aneurysm.

Eighty-five percent of arteriovenous malformations are located in the cerebral hemispheres, most commonly in the parieto-occipital regions. Subarachnoid hemorrhage may be one of the initial signs. Headaches, seizures, and intellectual and psychic disturbances are frequent symptoms. There may also be transient episodes of monocular blindness, photopsias, and transient homonymous hemianopias. The most common neuro-ophthalmologic complication of these arteriovenous malformations is homonymous hemianopia which is sometimes bilateral and causes "cerebral blindness."

The arteriovenous fistula of the internal carotid artery within the cavernous sinus, that is either traumatic (75%) or spontaneous (25%) does not result in a cavernous sinus syndrome. The most important sign is exophthalmos on the side of the fistula. Contralateral exophthalmos may follow in about one-third of the cases in several days or weeks. The exophthalmos may be pulsating and the pulsation is synchronous with the radial pulse. A characteristic bruit, which is synchronous with the pulse, can be heard with the stethoscope in the frontotemporal region or directly over the orbit. There may also be disturbances of motility including a sixth nerve paresis, and oculomotor paresis. This may result in ptosis as well as a mydriatic pupil which is fixed to light. There may be venous stasis which produces dilated conjunctival veins with ecchymosis, dilatation of the veins of the lids with edema of the lids, dilated and tortuous scleral veins, and dilated retinal veins with signs of retinal hemorrhage. There may also be evidence of papilledema which may evolve to optic atrophy. Initially, there is no loss of vision or visual field changes. These develop later, as does, occasionally, secondary glaucoma. This arteriovenous malformation must be differentiated from tumors of the orbit or a sphenoid ridge meningioma. Other tumors at the base of the skull, which produce a superior orbital fissure syndrome, must be considered. Tumors usually do not produce the marked venous congestion, pulsating exophthalmos as well as the bruit. However, a pulsating exophthalmos can be produced by aneurysms of the ophthalmic artery, an arteriovenous malformation within the orbit, or with a neurofibroma. Bilateral carotid angiography as well as orbital phlebography must be performed.

COMPLICATIONS OF ORAL CONTRACEPTIVES

Neuro-ophthalmologic complications have been reported in patients taking oral contraceptive agents. It is not yet known whether these complications represent the direct result of the administration of these drugs or whether they are merely incidental occurrences. The fact remains that there has been an increase in the number of women, between the ages of 20 to 45, taking the oral contraceptive agents, who present with the sudden onset of a homonymous hemianopia, hemiplegia, seizures, or increase in headaches. Since the administration of these drugs is accompanied by alterations in blood coagulation, it is possible that this may be a contributing factor in the production of these signs and symptoms. Other findings which are present in women taking the oral contraceptives include the syndrome of benign intracranial hypertension, diplopia, and optic neuritis. When there has been thrombosis of cerebral vessels, there may be permanent residuae and deaths have been reported.

PUPIL

Disturbances in pupillary function are very helpful in determining the presence of neuro-ophthalmologic disease as well as in its localization. Pupillary activity may reflect the integrity of many of the tracts of the central nervous system. Evaluation of the pupil has been discussed in the section on the examination of the unconscious patient. The differential diagnosis of the miotic and mydriatic pupil will be presented in Tables 7 and 8.

TABLE 7

DIFFERENTIAL DIAGNOSIS OF THE MIOTIC PUPIL

1. Physiologic anisocoria
2. Topical miotics
3. Iritis - acute or chronic
4. Horner's syndrome
5. Raeder's syndrome
6. Histamine cephalalgia (Horton's syndrome)
7. Argyll Robertson pupil
8. Cerebrovascular disease - thalamus, pons, medulla

268/ Neuro-Ophthalmologic Emergencies

```
┌─────────────────────────────────────────────────────────────┐
│                         TABLE 8                               │
│                                                               │
│      DIFFERENTIAL DIAGNOSIS OF THE MYDRIATIC PUPIL            │
│                                                               │
│   1.  Physiologic anisocoria                                  │
│   2.  Topical cycloplegics                                    │
│   3.  Aneurysm                                                │
│   4.  Diabetes                                                │
│   5.  Trauma - ocular, orbital, or intracranial               │
│   6.  Adie's syndrome                                         │
│   7.  Migraine                                                │
│   8.  Syphilis                                                │
│   9.  Glaucoma                                                │
│  10.  Posterior synechiae                                     │
│  11.  Aberrant regeneration of third nerve                    │
│  12.  Cerebrovascular disease - midbrain                      │
│  13.  Claude-Bernard syndrome                                 │
│  14.  General paresis                                         │
└─────────────────────────────────────────────────────────────┘
```

Afferent lesions in the visual pathways may produce either the amaurotic or the Marcus-Gunn pupil, depending upon the severity of the lesion. The presence of the Marcus-Gunn pupil is helpful in the diagnosis of optic nerve disease when the visual acuity is mildly impaired. The direct reaction to light will be normal, but when the light is moved from the normal eye to the impaired eye, the pupil will dilate under the influence of the light. This indicates a conduction defect anterior to the chiasm. Defects of the afferent tract will not produce anisocoria. Abnormalities of the pupil include the Argyll Robertson pupil as well as light-near dissociation of the pupils. Defects of the efferent tracts of the pupil can produce a Hutchinson pupil, which is a dilated pupil fixed to light and near, occurring in patients with increased intracranial pressure. This is produced by compression of the third cranial nerve against the dorsum sellae or the petroclinoid ligament, interrupting the efferent pathway to the pupil ipsilateral to the herniation of the uncus of the temporal lobe. This sign must be recognized rapidly and steps taken to remedy it. Adie's tonic pupil is also caused by an efferent abnormality. In the syndrome of aberrant regeneration of the third cranial nerve, the pupil constricts on adduction and dilates on abduction. This is found with an aneurysm, intracranial neoplasm, or following trauma. It has not been associated with diabetes.

Horner's syndrome may occur with brainstem disease, metastatic tumors or carcinoma of the lung (Pancoast's tumor). If damage to the sympathetic pathways occurs during early life, as with injury to the brachial plexus, heterochromia iridis may occur.

The fixed dilated pupil (Table 9) may be caused by midbrain damage secondary to vascular disease, neoplasms and infectious diseases. When the ventral portion of the midbrain is involved, usually there are associated neurologic defects involving the cerebral peduncles as well as the red nuclei. Damage to the third nerve from the interpeduncular fossa to the ciliary ganglion can produce a fixed dilated pupil. This can occur with aneurysms, neoplasms, meningitis, and a parasellar lesion or a sellar lesion.

TABLE 9

CAUSES OF A FIXED, DILATED PUPIL

1. Midbrain disease
2. Damage to third nerve from interpeduncular fossa to ciliary ganglion
3. Damage to ciliary ganglion or short ciliary nerves
4. Damage to iris

Involvement of the ciliary ganglion or short ciliary nerves, following a viral infection such as herpes zoster, and orbital trauma or tumor as well as choroidal trauma or tumor, can also produce the dilated fixed pupil. Blunt trauma to the globe may injure the ciliary plexus at the iris root. It must also be remembered that damage to the iris from inflammatory disease, posterior synechiae, a rise of intraocular pressure as well as traumatic iridoplegia and pharmacologic blockade can produce the fixed dilated pupil.

MIDBRAIN

Ocular manifestations of midbrain dysfunction affect predominantly vertical gaze. The vertical gaze impairment may first manifest itself as vertical nystagmus. The midbrain may be affected by vascular disease, trauma, inflammation, tumors, and degenerative diseases.

Parinaud's syndrome consists of paralysis of vertical gaze, affecting upward gaze first, and downward gaze later, pupillary areflexia to light, and weakness of convergence.

The presence of a bilateral oculomotor paralysis with quadriplegia, commencing in the upper extremities, indicates disease of the interpeduncular fossa. This may be caused by aneurysms or mass lesions involving the oculomotor nerves and cerebral peduncles.

Patients with involvement of the medial longitudinal fasciculus may complain of diplopia, as well as oscillopsia (perception of objects moving). The patient may not have any subjective complaints but objective findings indicate involvement of this structure, an internuclear ophthalmoplegia. Internuclear ophthalmoplegia consists of weakness of adduction in one eye combined with nystagmus of the abducting eye on attempted lateral gaze. Impairment of convergence implicates a midbrain lesion and thus an anterior internuclear ophthalmoplegia. Preservation of convergence and weakness of abduction denotes involvement of the pons or posterior internuclear ophthalmoplegia. Unilateral involvement of the medial longitudinal fasciculus is usually secondary to vascular disease of the brainstem.

Ptosis has been recorded in approximately 60% of patients with an intracranial aneurysm. The ptosis is usually unilateral and is attributed to pressure upon the fibers of the levator palpebri in the

intracranial course of the third nerve. A diabetic ophthalmoplegia may be the presenting sign of diabetes mellitus. The pupil is
spared in about 90% of the patients. The ophthalmoplegia with diabetes mellitus usually recovers in approximately two to three
months and recurrences are not common.

In any patient with unexplained ptosis, consideration must be given
to the presence of myasthenia gravis. Patients usually present with
ptosis involving first one lid and then the other.

Oculomotor palsies producing ptosis can occur following head trauma as well as direct or indirect trauma to the orbit. The ptosis of
Horner's syndrome is associated with a miotic pupil. Moreover, it
should be remembered that a wide pupil on the same side as the
ptosis indicates disease of the oculomotor nerve, whereas a miotic
pupil on the same side as the ptosis indicates a lesion of the sympathetic nervous system.

Diplopia may be produced by defects in function of the third, fourth,
or sixth cranial nerves. Moreover, disease of the neuromuscular
junction, such as myasthenia gravis, can also produce double vision.
There must be an asymmetric defect in innervation of the extraocular muscles in order to produce diplopia.

POSTERIOR FOSSA

Bilateral lesions of the pontine paramedian reticular formation at
the level of the abducens nuclei produce paralysis of all horizontal
eye movements. There is also lack of the reflex ocular deviation
stimulated by caloric irrigation. Destructive unilateral lesions of
the pontine paramedian reticular formation cause weakness of
horizontal gaze towards the side of the lesion or a gaze-paretic
jerk nystagmus towards the same side.

Ocular "bobbing" refers to intermittent rapid downward eye movements with return of the eyes to the primary position and indicates
pathology in the pons.

Defective function of the vestibular nuclei produces a rapid, jerk-
type horizontal nystagmus with a prominent rotary component, with
the fast phase towards the side of the lesion.

Lesions of the frontal lobe can produce deviation of the eyes towards the side of the lesion with lack of voluntary eye movements
to the contralateral side. However, when the head is passively rotated (doll's head phenomena) and with caloric irrigation, the eyes
will deviate to the contralateral side. Caloric responses and the
oculocephalic maneuver are depressed, with lesions involving the
pontine paramedian reticular formation in the pons when the abducens nucleus is also involved. With lesions of the brainstem, the
eyes are usually in the midline unless a superimposed sixth nerve
palsy exists and then an esodeviation with uncrossed diplopia will
exist.

Diplopia is usually not present when there is weakness of conjugate eye movement associated with supranuclear lesions, but cranial nerve palsies and diplopia are frequently found with disease of the midbrain and pons, cranial nerves, orbit, and extraocular muscles (Tables 10-14).

In the presence of cerebral lesions hemianopic field defects and depressed optokinetic responses will be found on rotating the tape towards the side of the lesion; however, in brainstem lesions the abnormal optokinetic response is elicited when the tape is rotated away from the side of the abnormality.

The nystagmus associated with disease of the vestibular nuclei is usually accompanied by nausea, vomiting, and tinnitus. It is horizontal with a marked rotary component. Vestibular nystagmus also varies in amplitude and frequency with the position of the head.

Vertical nystagmus, in the absence of dilantin, phenobarbital, or other sedative medication, indicates disease of the posterior fossa. The fast phase is directed upward. When vertical nystagmus manifests the rapid phase downward, dysfunction of the medulla or high cervical cord usually exists. However, this may also occur with disease of the midbrain, but can be accompanied by the rapid phase being upward as well.

The fifth and seventh cranial nerves are involved in disease of the pons and medulla. Lesions of the pons may thus produce pressure on the fifth, sixth, and seventh cranial nerves, resulting in loss of the corneal reflex, sixth nerve palsy, and a peripheral type of seventh nerve palsy. A differential diagnosis of isolated sixth nerve palsies is found in Table 13.

The hallmark of disease of the pons is the existence of multiple cranial nerve palsies.

The ocular manifestations of cerebellar disease are related to defective ocular movements as well as increased intracranial pressure. Acute lesions of the cerebellar hemispheres will cause a gaze paresis or palsy and conjugate ocular deviation to the contralateral side with impairment of eye movements to the side of the lesion.

The eye movement disorders of cerebellar disease include ocular dysmetria, ocular flutter, skew deviation, and nystagmus. Nystagmus is usually present in more than 50% of the patients with cerebellar mass lesions. It is a gaze-paretic nystagmus toward the side of the lesion. The nystagmus associated with disease of the cerebellum may represent brainstem dysfunction.

Papilledema is a frequent manifestation of cerebellar mass lesions. Increased intracranial pressure may produce disturbances in cranial nerve function. About 20% of the patients with cerebellar tumors will manifest weakness of the lateral rectus or decreased corneal sensation.

Gliomas of the pons and ependymomas can produce multiple cranial nerve palsies in association with ataxia, pyramidal tract signs, sensory loss and horizontal and vertical nystagmus with conjugate gaze palsies. These signs can be produced similarly by the medulloblastoma and the hemiangioblastoma. The cranial nerve signs with a brainstem tumor are usually bilateral.

The supraorbital and infraorbital branches of the trigeminal nerve may be injured by trauma leading to numbness in the forehead and infraorbital region. Injury to the infraorbital nerve can produce numbness of the cheek, upper lip, and upper teeth. This can be found with fractures of the maxillary bone as well as fractures of the floor of the orbit. Involvement of the trigeminal nerve can occur with lesions in the cavernous sinus as well as in injuries in the brainstem when there is accompanying evidence of multiple cranial nerve palsies. A partial facial nerve palsy can result from soft tissue injury to the face with edema, causing involvement of the peripheral branches of the facial nerve. The facial nerve can be injured with fractures of the petrous and mastoid portions of the temporal bone.

TABLE 10

DIFFERENTIAL DIAGNOSIS OF UNILATERAL, ISOLATED OCULOMOTOR PARALYSIS

1. Aneurysm
2. Diabetes
3. Neuropathy
4. Neoplasm
5. Trauma
6. Migraine
7. Temporal arteritis
8. Myasthenia gravis
9. Nasopharyngeal tumor
10. Infectious mononucleosis
11. Syphilis
12. Carotid-cavernous fistula
13. A-V malformation

TABLE 11

DIFFERENTIAL DIAGNOSIS OF UNILATERAL, ISOLATED TROCHLEAR NERVE PARALYSIS

1. Trauma
   a. Orbit
   b. Head
2. Arteriosclerosis and hypertension
3. Diabetes
4. Multiple sclerosis
5. Sickle-cell anemia

TABLE 12

DIFFERENTIAL DIAGNOSIS OF DIPLOPIA

1. Fracture of orbit
2. Orbital hematoma
3. Trauma to extraocular muscles in orbit
4. Subluxation of lens
5. Macular edema
6. Third nerve palsy (orbital or intracranial)
7. Fourth nerve palsy (orbital or intracranial)
8. Sixth nerve palsy (orbital or intracranial)
9. Multiple cranial nerve palsies
10. Myasthenia gravis
11. Thyroid ophthalmopathy
12. Temporal arteritis
13. Tolosa-Hunt syndrome
14. Herpes zoster
15. Multiple sclerosis
16. Decompensation of existing phoria to tropia

TABLE 13

DIFFERENTIAL DIAGNOSIS OF UNILATERAL,
ISOLATED SIXTH NERVE PALSY

1. Arteriosclerosis and hypertension
2. Viral - children
3. Neoplasm
4. Increased intracranial pressure
5. Head trauma
6. Diabetes
7. Multiple sclerosis
8. Myasthenia gravis
9. Gradenigo's syndrome
10. Meningitis
11. Syphilis
12. Wernicke's encephalopathy
13. Following dental injections
14. Following lumbar puncture
15. Arteriovenous fistula (carotid-cavernous)

Trigeminal neuralgia (tic douloureux) is characterized by recurrent episodes of sharp, stabbing pains in the distribution of one or more branches of the fifth cranial nerve. The second or third divisions are most frequently involved, the maxillary branch slightly more than the mandibular. The ophthalmic division is affected in less than 5% of the cases. However, pain which has been originally confined to one division may spread to involve other divisions. There is no objective sensory loss and motor function of the nerve is normal. The best treatment for trigeminal neuralgia is Tegretol, 200 mg, two to five times a day.

BRAIN TUMORS

Ocular signs can be observed in about 50% of the patients with brain tumors. These ocular manifestations may be the initial complaints in the early stages. In about 60% of the patients with brain tumors, papilledema is found. The presence of characteristic ocular signs may enable the physician to localize accurately the region of the brain involved. In addition to papilledema there may be mental changes and visual field defects. The visual field defects which occur in patients with brain tumors include a general and concentric constriction, unilateral sector-shaped abnormalities secondary to compression of the optic nerve, bitemporal field defects including bitemporal quadrantanopias, asymmetric bitemporal hemianopias, or quadrantanopias, amaurosis of one eye associated with temporal hemianopia of the other eye, central or centrocaecal scotomas and homonymous field defects. Homonymous quadrantanopias can be produced by tumors of the temporal lobe when a superior homonymous quadrantanopia exists. Tumors of the parietal lobe produce an inferior homonymous quadrantanopia and tumors of the occipital lobe produce complete homonymous hemianopias with marked congruity.

INFECTION

Ocular signs and symptoms may be produced by meningitis and encephalitis. Meningitis is diagnosed, usually, on the basis of meningeal signs including severe headaches, stiff neck, photophobia, eyeball tenderness and pain on ocular motion, pain in the back on straight leg raising, and low back pain. The abducens nerve and oculomotor nerves may be involved, producing ptosis or extraocular muscle palsies with pupillary changes and anisocoria. Papilledema may also be present. A superimposed uveitis can ensue. A lumbar puncture should be performed and a culture and sensitivity, as well as an immediate Gram stain, in order to commence the use of appropriate antibiotics. Tuberculous meningitis can also produce signs of extraocular muscle palsies, increased intracranial pressure, as well as impairment of optic nerve function. Encephalitis can produce signs which are most characteristic of involvement of the midbrain, pons, and medulla, or cerebral hemisphere disease with marked mental changes as well. Encephalitis can follow measles, mumps, chicken pox, or small pox vaccination.

Brain abscesses produce similar ocular signs and symptoms as other space-occupying lesions such as brain tumors. The most common location of abscesses include the temporal lobe and the cerebellum, secondary to extension from an otitis media.

FUNCTIONAL VS. ORGANIC VISUAL IMPAIRMENT

It is frequently important to differentiate between a functional and organic ocular defect. The presence of a Marcus-Gunn pupillary phenomenon indicates optic nerve or retinal pathology. The Marcus-Gunn pupillary sign is not present in amblyopia, malingering, or hysteria. Examination of the visual acuity, using the phoropter, is helpful in differentiating organic from functional-impaired visual acuity. One can manipulate the lenses before both eyes simultaneously and, thus, by intermittently impairing vision of the good eye, determine that the so-called "bad eye" is being used. Examination of the visual fields is important since it is the rare patient who understands that 10 degrees of visual field covers an area with twice the diameter at 2 meters than it does at one meter. In addition, a specific target is only half as effective visually when it is twice as far from the patient. The hysterical or malingering patient will usually not complain of a central scotoma. Occasionally, it is possible to determine the malingerer by having a chart with a 20/70 letter on top. He may read only the top letters and claim inability to read further. Often an individual who refuses to read beyond 20/200 will read small print when he is suddenly presented with a reading chart. If an individual maintains that one eye is defective to the extent that it cannot be used in reading, he is asked to read and suddenly a plus 10 sphere is placed in front of the sound eye. If the reading continues, it is obvious that the suspected eye is being used. A prism of 10 prism diopters, base out, may be placed in front of the suspected eye while the patient is reading only with the sound eye. If the eye being examined has visual acuity, it will turn inward and, when the prism is removed, will move outward to maintain binocular vision. If the prism is placed base up or base down before the suspected eye while the individual is reading aloud, and the suspected eye is amaurotic or highly amblyopic, the reading will be continued without any problems. If the vision in the suspected eye is nearly normal, there will be immediate difficulty in reading or it may be impossible for him to do so.

TABLE 14

BILATERAL OPHTHALMOPLEGIA OF SUDDEN ONSET

1. Brainstem vascular accident, basilar artery syndrome
2. Wernicke's disease, Leigh's disease
3. Pituitary apoplexy - hemorrhage
4. Miller-Fisher syndrome - Viral Guillain-Barre syndrome
5. Myasthenia gravis
6. Bulbar poliomyelitis
7. Diphtheria, botulism
8. Tuberculosis and lues

BIBLIOGRAPHY

1. Bender, M. B. (ed.): The Approach to Diagnosis in Modern Neurology. Grune and Stratton, New York, 1967.

2. Cogan, D. G.: Neurology of the Ocular Muscles, 2nd ed. Charles C Thomas, Springfield, 1972.

3. Cogan, D. G.: Neurology of the Visual System. Charles C Thomas, Springfield, 1970.

4. Huber, A.: Trans. (Blodi, F. C.): Eye Symptoms in Brain Tumors, 2nd ed. Grune and Stratton, New York, 1961.

5. Kestenbaum, A.: Clinical Methods of Neuro-Ophthalmologic Examination, 2nd ed. Grune and Stratton, New York, 1961.

6. Merritt, H. H.: A Textbook of Neurology, 5th ed. Lea and Febiger, Philadelphia, 1973.

7. Plum, F. and Posner, J. B.: The Diagnosis of Stupor and Coma, 2nd ed. Davis, Philadelphia, 1972.

8. Scheie, H. G. and Albert, D. M.: Adler's Textbook of Ophthalmology. Saunders, Philadelphia, 1969.

9. Toole, J. F. and Patel, A. N.: Cerebrovascular Disorders, 2nd ed. McGraw-Hill, New York, 1974.

10. Walsh, F. B. and Hoyt, W. F.: Clinical Neuro-Ophthalmology, 3rd ed. Williams and Wilkins, Baltimore, 1969.